12-88

Leo —

Many thanks to you and the staff for your assistance with this book.

Al

**Home Health Aides:
How to Manage
The People Who Help You**

For information about ordering copies of this publication, please see the last page of this book.

Home Health Aides:
How to Manage The People Who Help You

Alfred H. DeGraff

Editorial Assistance: Margaret Short-DeGraff

Saratoga Access Publications

HOME HEALTH AIDES: HOW TO MANAGE THE PEOPLE WHO HELP YOU. Copyright 1988 by Alfred H. DeGraff. All rights reserved. Printed in the United States of America. No part of this book may be used or reproduced in any manner whatsoever (to include making copies for instructional applications or handouts) without written permission, except in the case of brief quotations embodied in critical articles or reviews. For information write Saratoga Access Publications, P.O. Box 2346, Clifton Park, New York 12065.

Saratoga Access Publications specializes in materials which teach skills of independent living. Written inquiries are welcome from unpublished authors and agencies. Please, no telephone inquiries. Please initially request an inquiry application form; unsolicited abstracts and manuscripts can be neither reviewed nor returned.

Cataloging Data

88-92446

ISBN 0-9621106-0-4

First Edition
10 9 8 7 6 5 4 3 2 1

For information about ordering copies of this publication, please see the last page of this book.

Dedication to My Previous PCAs

Throughout this handbook, you will find many first names randomly used in examples and illustrations. Each name which appears, however, is the actual name of one of the many PCAs whom I have recruited, interviewed, trained, and with whom I have parted ways during my 20-plus years of using personal help.

Each PCA has taught me something about being a better manager. I have learned from strategies which worked well, as well as from those which failed miserably. With some PCAs I am still Christmas card friends, some others left owing me money or my possessions, and at least one is no longer living.

Regardless, Previous PCAs, I'm grateful for the help and management skills which you gave me. If you spot your first name in this handbook, know that some contribution which you gave my management experience is now benefitting other PCA managers who are using this text throughout the world!

Table of Contents

Preface..13
Acknowledgements...16

∎ Introduction
Why this Handbook is Unique and Important to You..........21

Definition of Terms to be Used in this Book........................24
 -PCA, Nurse, Aide, Nursing Assistant, Nurses Aide, Home Health Aide, Personal Care Aide or Attendant, Homemaker, Housekeeper, Household Maintenance, Domestic Cook, Sitter, Companion, Transportation Driver

∎ Section I: Why Should You Learn Management Skills?
1) Rights for You and the PCA..29

2) Two Approaches to "Aide/Attendant Instruction & Manuals"...32
 -Training the <u>Aides</u> for Those Who Receive Assistance
 -Training <u>Those Who Require Assistance</u> to be Able to Independently Manage the Aides Whom They Use

3) Why Should You Learn to Manage the Help You Use?......36
 -The 6 Freedoms:
 -Freedom to directly control the type, quality, and schedule of aides -- and to change aides -- whenever necessary
 -Freedom from being dependent upon aide pools or referral-agency lists, and the consequent ability to geographically relocate wherever and whenever necessary
 -Freedom from having to use agency or college campus aide/attendant training services
 -Freedom from having to pay the high hourly administrative rates to professional home health aide agencies if one is not eligible for 3rd party funding
 -Freedom from having to use parents or relatives as aides
 -Freedom from having to use a spouse as an aide, or sole aide

4) The 3 Management Situations:
   Which One Applies to You?..46
   -You have all the abilities required for managing those who provide you assistance
   -You have the emotional and mental abilities, however lack physical, visual, or verbal abilities for some management tasks
   -You are not able or willing to manage those who provide you assistance

▪ Section II: Strategies for Being a Good Manager
5) The Top 10 Reasons Why PCAs Quit & Are Fired..............63

6) Settings in Which You Use Help...67
   -Acute Care Hospital
   -Rehabilitation Hospital
   -Transitional & Residential Independent Living Center
   -Nursing Home or Infirmary
   -Private Housing
   -College Residence Hall or Voc-Tech/Campus Area Housing
   -Day or Evening Travel
   -Overnight Travel

7) Types of Help & the Services Which Each Provider Performs..92
   -Health Professionals Working at Institutions
   -Agency-Provided Health Professionals in Your Home
   -Health Professionals Whom You Employ in Your Home
   -Comparisons: Should You Use Agency-Provided or Personally Recruited Help in Your Home?

8) Qualities and Strategies of a Good Manager...................115

9) Passive, Aggressive, & Assertive:
   Which Style is Best for Stating Needs?..........................122

10) Job Expectations..129
    -The PCA's Expectations of You
    -Your Expectations of the PCA

Table of Contents

11) The Favorable Physical Work Environment 139
    -A Clean and Pleasant Work Area
    -An Efficient Layout of Each Work Area
    -A Sufficient Inventory of Supplies
    -Prescription Medical Equipment: Stocking the Supplies and Tools of Preventative Maintenance

■ **Section III: Identifying & Dividing My Needs for Assistance**

12) Abusing Help with Inappropriate Requests 155

13) 3 Types of Activities Which Qualify for PCA Help 157
    -Request Primarily Physical Assistance
    -3 Types of Activities Which Qualify for PCA Help
    -4 Ways to Request Help from PCAs

14) Making A Master List of Your Needs for Assistance 165
    -Advantages to Making a List
    -Steps to Follow in Making Your List
    -An Example

15) Dividing Needs with More Than One PCA 172
    -Advantages to Dividing
    -When Dividing is Wise & Unwise
    -Strategies for Dividing Your Needs

■ **Section IV: Paying Salaries & Taxes**

16) Methods for Paying PCAs 185
    -Volunteer PCA Help: Don't Over-Use It or Rely On It
    -Paying PCAs with Appreciation & Salary: Strategies for Expressing Appreciation

17) Salaries: Determining Salary Rates
    & Merit Increases 192
    -3 Options for Using Starting Salaries
     & Merit Increases
    -Starting Salary Rates
    -Merit Increase Rates & Schedules

18) Monetary Salaries: Cash, Noncash, or Both 198
    -Cash Salaries
    -Personal-Budget Funding for Cash Salaries
    -3rd-Party Funding for Cash Salaries
    -Noncash Salaries

19) Tax Obligations for a PCA Employer............................210
   -Kinds of Employees Whom You Directly Employ
   -Knowing Your Obligations, When Paying Cash Wages
   -Knowing Your Obligations, When Paying Noncash Wages
   -Record Keeping Strategies

20) Medical Deductions & Credits for PCA Employers......222
   -Deducting PCA Cash & Noncash Salaries
   -Tax Credits for PCA Services
   -Services as Medical or Business-Related Deductions

21) A List of IRS Tax Publications for PCA Employers......226

∎ Section V: Recruiting, Interviewing, Training, & Parting with Help

22) Creating a Job Description for PCAs............................229
   -The Importance of a Job Description
   -Parts of a Job Description
   -Job Description Examples

23) Residence Locations for a PCA......................................246
   -As a Roommate
   -In the Same Living Area
   -In the Same Building
   -Within the Nearby Neighborhood
   -Using a Variety of PCAs to Advantage

24) Sources for Recruiting PCAs..251
   -Referrals from Current PCAs
   -Previous PCA Applicants or Employees
   -Home Health Aide Agencies
   -Nearby College Campus
   -Surrounding Community
   -Local Medical Facilities
   -Disability Organizations in a Campus or Community
   -Employment Agency

25) Methods for Recruiting PCAs......................................261
   -Some Secrets of Advertising
   -Newspaper Ads and Newsletter Notices
   -Posters and Index Card Notices
   -Expressing the PCA Position by Word-of-Mouth
    or by Telephone

Table of Contents

26) Interviewing, Screening, & Hiring Prospective PCAs..279
    - Objectives for Interviewing & Screening
    - Applicant Traits to Favor and Avoid
    - Interview Observation Skills from Sherlock Holmes
    - Step-by-Step Procedure

27) Training and Ongoing Management............................304
    - Adopting the Qualities of a Good Manager
    - Becoming Organized
    - Providing Clear Instruction to New PCAs
    - Providing Good Ongoing Management to PCAs

28) Predicting, Recognizing, & Resolving PCA Problems..313
    - Correcting Simple Performance Problems
    - Signs of a Healthy Job Relationship
    - Symptoms of an Unhealthy Job Relationship
    - Possible Reasons Behind Negative Symptoms
    - Steps in Resolving These and Other Problems
    - When PCA Problems Cannot Be Resolved, Prepare to Part Ways

29) Parting Ways from a PCA...323
    - Depression About a Departing PCA is Common
    - The Simple Facts Behind a PCA Departure
    - Steps to Accepting the Resignation from a PCA
    - Steps to Firing a PCA

30) 10 Top Guidelines for Maximum Independent Living..331

    Your Personal Management Notes:
    What Has Worked for You, and What Has Not..............341

    How to Order Copies of this Book................................345

Preface

"Give me a fish

and I eat for a day,

Teach me to fish

and I eat for a lifetime!" **

- author unknown

The morning of July 4, 1967 was hot and muggy. I was 18 years old, had graduated from high school just a few days before, and I was working for the summer on Martha's Vineyard, Massachusetts.

The Vineyard is a well-known resort island, about 7 miles off Cape Cod. As any island, it is surrounded by beautiful ocean beaches.

That 4th of July was a holiday for me from my clerking in a clothing store, and I sprang out of bed and pulled on my swim trunks. I was in great physical shape and thoroughly enjoyed bicycling the 5 miles to the Vineyard's South Beach. I had planned to spend the day tanning, swimming, and boosting my social life.

After an hour of tanning, munching on apples from the local A & P, and listening to the AM-radio '60s rock of WBZ (Boston) and WABC (Manhattan), it was time to cool off in the Atlantic. Around 10:00 that morning, I paddled my feet through the hot sand and climbed up onto a concrete pier which nosed out into the crashing, cold surf. Standing tall at the front edge of the pier, I looked out toward the huge waves rolling toward my toes.

** The spirit behind learning as many independent living skills as possible, and minimizing one's dependence on others.

As many of us teenagers had done on previous days, I curled my toes tightly around the front edge of the pier, leaned forward like a cat about to spring toward a mouse, and dove head-first into a fat, incoming wave.

That simple dive would change the rest of my life.

I felt the cold, refreshing splash of salty ocean against my face as I entered the water...and then I heard a "snap." Regardless of the large outward size of that wave, I had apparently dived the 15 vertical feet downward into low tide. My forehead hit the sandy ocean floor, my neck snapped at the C-5/6 level, and my body was instantly and painlessly paralyzed below the level of my broken neck.

Another sun bather saw me floating face-down and before I had used my initial deep breath of air, I was pulled from the water. Still very conscious and cracking jokes as a probable defense against my body's traumatic state of shock, I was flown by air ambulance to Massachusetts General Hospital.

My new lifestyle had begun.

My mother temporarily left her upstate New York home and moved into a summer sublet among "all those hippies" on Boston's Beacon Hill. With patience only mothers have, her daily stays at my hospital bedside provided the essential psychological support that my adjustment required. Thank you, Mom, I love you.

My medical situation stabilized within 2 1/2 months and I then transferred to Sunnyview Hospital in upstate New York for an additional 11 months of rehabilitation.

I was then, and remain, paralyzed below the chest with neither motor control nor sensation. Medically, I am classified a "quadriplegic," because all four limbs are affected; typical of other "quads," I have partial use of my hands and arms.

This situation may sound depressing to able-bodied folks, however I discovered early that I could minimize depression simply by avoiding thoughts about my inabilities. I learned

Preface 15

to avoid teasing myself with wanting to do things which are beyond my new set of abilities.

Instead, I needed to concentrate on my abilities, set some realistic goals, and get back on life's track. The first step was to learn all I could about living as independently as possible from my cabinet of "rehabilitation advisors" at the hospital.

As for so many types of physical disabilities, the objective for my in-patient "rehab" was not a cure back to "able-bodiedness." Instead, it meant receiving authoritative advice from highly trained medical professionals on making the most of the physical abilities remaining from a disability. Surgeons, rehab physicians, physical and occupational therapists, social workers, and psychologists each had separate areas of expertise for training people with various disabilities in accommodating their limitations.

However, there is one serious void which no medical authority typically addresses in much detail.

Most people who have significant physical disabilities will require a lifetime of routine physical assistance from others in order to accomplish daily activities. Some folks require very little help; some need a lot. These activities can include personal care, household upkeep, and pursuing goals of education, career, recreation, leisure...and just plain "living life to its fullest."

Typically, there is no health professional -- or even reference text -- which addresses how to manage the people who provide that physical assistance. Most "attendant books" teach <u>attendants or aides who provide help</u> in ways to perform nursing procedures, but very few teach <u>the individual who uses help</u> how to recruit, interview, instruct, salary, and otherwise manage the people who provide that help.

Many hospitals assume that home health aide agencies will provide plenty of employed and well trained aides, and that the dependent patient will have no need to learn or practice any management skills.

This is a poor assumption.

In truth, there are several reasons outlined in this book why agencies often cannot meet the needs of many clients. Consequently, an increasing population of people who use home health aides is directly recruiting the aides it uses. These direct recruiters who do not use agencies need a wide range of management skills.

Even the individual who does use trained, agency aides requires skills in instructing, supervising, and keeping happy those aides around his/her unique needs for help.

In order to be active and to maximize independence, people with a disability must be in control of the quality, type, and scheduling of help that they receive. If they are not in control of these factors and the people who provide assistance, then they have lost the freedom to choose their own lifestyle.

For over 20 years now, I have hired and managed the attendants and aides who have helped me. As outlined on the back cover of this book, the ability to hire and use help in a wide variety of settings has enabled me to enjoy a life rich in education, careers, and travel...even though I remain 80% paralyzed.

This is the only complete handbook which enables <u>people who use physical help</u> to be in control of that help, and consequently to retain their freedom and to be active in the lifestyle they choose.

Alfred H. "Skip" DeGraff
Saratoga Springs, New York
1988

Acknowledgements

My previous, 38-page book on a similar topic, "Attendants and Attendees: A Guidebook of Helpful Hints," was published in 1979 by the College and University Personnel Association, Washington, D.C. I am grateful for the assistance of Carole Sturgis and Janet Long, formerly consultants to CUPA, for their assistance with that publication.

This new edition contains contributions from Judy Ameen Wilchynski, Carolyn Wojcik, and Ricky Hoyt. Definitions and concepts of the terms passive, aggressive, and assertive came from "Assert Yourself!, How to Be Your Own Person," Merna Dee and John P. Galassi (Human Services Press, New York 1977). Quotations in chapter 30 marked with an asterisk (*) are from signer-songwriter Barry Manilow, spoken at the end of his 1987 and 1988 concerts, and appearing in his book, "Sweet Life," Barry Manilow (McGraw Hill, New York 1987).

Most of all, I appreciate the assistance of my wife, Margaret Short-DeGraff. Peggy has provided routine encouragement and advice during my years of writing this text, and then assisted with copyediting after it was written. She is widely published in journals and books. I am very proud of her.

Additional thanks go to the Skidmore Computer Services at Skidmore College and to Bonnie Rieser, Boston.

Statement of Lack of Gender Bias

Throughout the design and writing of this text, the author has carefully guarded against any gender bias by using gender nouns, pronouns, and possessives randomly and in approximate equal frequency.

Introduction

Why This Book is Unique and Important to You

Definition of "PCA" and Other Terms Used in This Book

Why This Handbook is Unique and Important to You

The number of people who require medical and physical assistance from others, as well as the market of people who are willing to provide that assistance, are growing at a fast rate. With this growth in both service recipients and providers is a similar increase in the need for a complete handbook which instructs you, the actual recipient of assistance, in how to manage that assistance from others.

This is the only, step-by-step reference handbook which extensively instructs recipients of assistance how to be in control of the help which they use.

If you require assistance, you might use it while living alone at home, with relatives or a spouse, at a college or university campus, during daily meetings and appointments, for long-distance travel, or in a health institution of a hospital, rehabilitation center, independent living center, or nursing home. The requirement for assistance can be temporary, while you recuperate from a temporary illness or disability, or from a current medical viewpoint the requirement might be termed "life-long." Assistance is used everyday by children, teen-agers, college students, those employed in careers, those pursuing cultural and recreational activities, and seniors.

> Whether you use aides from a home health agency or directly employ your own, you need management skills

You might hire assistance through a professional agency, or directly recruit and manage the assistance which you are using. Funding for the help might come from your own personal budget or from a funding source such as an insurance company or a government program.

It is becoming common for private individuals who require assistance to directly recruit, interview and screen, hire, train, supervise, and otherwise manage the help which they use. For others who are either unable or unwilling to independently manage help, the supervision and management first might come from family members who directly employ the assistance for the recipient, or secondly from health institutions or home health agencies which professionally employ the assistance.

This second alternative for those unable or unwilling to manage help comes from professional home health aide agencies. These agencies often recruit, employ, train, and schedule aides for those who need their assistance. However, even when using well-trained aides, the recipient of assistance usually finds that he must have some management skills for instructing an agency's aide in the fine details of the particular duties which he requires.

People who provide care and physical assistance for others "come in all shapes and sizes." They can be full- or part-time employees of a health institution, a home health aide agency, or a government agency, or they can be directly employed by the individual who actually receives the assistance.

As discussed later in this book, using volunteers for day-to-day, routine needs for which one is completely dependent for assistance from others is rarely successful and not advised. However, individuals who require physical assistance for other types of needs do find that they need and successfully use very short-term, one-shot assistance from volunteers.

As contrasted with long-term, routine needs in one's home, there are frequently brief, one-time needs which one has while independently using public facilities for educational, career, religious, cultural, and recreational activities. This quick help from strangers can include holding open doors, retrieving out-of-reach shelf items in stores or libraries, and carrying packages to a car or van. Providing short-distance assistance to wheelchair users is also required when sudden equipment breakdowns occur, a brief push is needed up a ramp or incline, or when parking lot snow makes routinely independent mobility impossible.

Those who provide assistance can be of either sex, almost any age, and have any combination of personal backgrounds and personality traits. They will have a number of reasons for wishing to provide assistance -- usually honorable, however occasionally not so honorable.

Why This Handbook is Unique and Important 23

Finally, those who provide assistance might be formally trained and certified in their line of work, not formally trained but experienced from having learned-on-the-job ("roads" scholars!), or lacking both training and previous experience but willing to learn while working for you.

Regardless of the "shape or size" or degree of previous training and experience, each provider who assists you will have at least one key request on first meeting you or the family member who represents you, "Please tell me what particular needs for assistance you have, and how and on what schedule you want me to provide that help."

For this and numerous other daily situations, you -- the actual recipient of services -- must have the skills to at least instruct, manage, and supervise the help which you use. If you directly employ the help which you use, you will require many skills in addition to these basics.

Definition of "PCA" & Other Terms to Be Used in this Book

PCA

This abbreviation is used by many groups and has acquired the two meanings of Personal Care Attendant and Personal Care Aide.

This term has been chosen for frequent use throughout this book, in the interest of brevity, clarity, and consequent ease to the readership, to refer to all types of assistants who provide physical help of any personal nature.

In this book, the term "PCA" can refer to a nurse, nursing assistant, home health aide, personal care aide or attendant, companion, sitter, homemaker, household maintenance, housekeeper, transportation driver, domestic cook, or other provider of similar personal assistance.

Nurse

Refers to someone with extensive medical training who expects to perform primarily medically-related procedures, as contrasted with household chores which are often performed by aides and certainly performed by housekeepers and other specialists.

> For ease of readership, the term "PCA" will be used throughout this book to refer to all types of assistants

Aide

also Nursing Assistant or Nurses Aide (often while working in a health facility), or Health Aide, Home Health Aide, Personal Care Aide or Attendant (often while working in a private home)

Refers to someone who provides assistance of primarily a medical nature, but which can include household duties, especially when directly employed by the private individual receiving the assistance.

Definition of Terms to Be Used in this Book

An aide has usually completed some degree of formal training if they are or have been employed by an agency or institution. This training probably consisted of textbook and classroom instruction followed by direct supervision and examination of their initial hours of providing care by a nurse-supervisor.

When employed by an agency or institution, the ongoing care provided by aides is directed and indirectly supervised by a nurse. When employed directly by a private individual in a home setting, the care is directed and supervised by the private individual who is being assisted or their representative. Aides who have received formal training and who are or have been employed by an agency or institution are often willing to earn extra salary by working beyond their agency or institutional hours directly for private individuals.

Homemaker
Housekeeper
Household Maintenance
Domestic Cook
Sitter
Companion
Transportation Driver

Refers to someone who provides assistance of household coordination or management, house cleaning, maintenance (repairs, lawn and landscape care, snow removal), cooking, companionship, or vehicular driving.

If this individual has been referred by a health institution or referral agency, they have probably received some degree of training which can range from a briefing about job responsibilities and interpersonal relations to extensive formal training and supervised initial experience.

Section I

Why Should You Learn Management Skills?

1) Rights for You and the PCA

2) Two Approaches to "Aide/Attendant Instruction & Manuals"

3) Why Should You Learn to Manage the Help You Use?

4) The 3 Management Situations: Which One Applies to You?

1. Rights for You and the PCA

Did you know that you, as a PCA employer, have certain rights on which you should be able to depend? Your need for physical assistance from others does not mean that you must lead a "second class life." On the flip side, however, have you ever considered that the PCAs you employ also have rights? They are not slaves who, because of a paycheck, are owned by their employer.

Here are the 2 lists published for the 1st time from informal polls of a number of PCA employers and PCA employees. All agree that most model PCA managers and most top-notch PCAs are those who routinely respect the rights of each other.

You -- the recipient of assistance -- have the right...

1) To interview, screen, and select the type and an adequate number of PCAs to assist you,

2) To select and assign the specific duties with which you need assistance, and to then receive communications which are delivered in a clear, direct, assertive manner which is neither weakly passive nor abusively aggressive,

3) To train PCAs to assist you in using methods which are safe, efficient, and which you prefer,

4) To schedule PCA assistance around a time structure that enables you to meet educational, career, and other timely responsibilities of the full life which you choose,

5) To maintain control over the quality and dependability of assistance which you receive,

> The single, most important factor toward long and happy employer-employee relationships is a respect for the rights of each other

6) To receive respect and dignity as an individual who, regardless of physical impairments, has a mind which is

fully capable of knowing your needs, making decisions, and managing the physical assistance which your body requires,

7) To receive confidentiality and privacy from PCAs for your personal thoughts, values, beliefs, relationships, and activities regardless of the required physical presence of the PCAs who assist you,

8) To security for your living quarters, personal possessions, food, medications, and financial assets,

9) To live life to its fullest in the manner and degree of social mainstream and independence which you choose, and

10) To fire and replace PCAs who do not respect these rights.

The PCA who assists you has the right...

1) To initially receive a clear, well-defined set of expected duties and time schedule, and to receive requests with an appropriate advance notice for any additional duties or schedule changes,

2) To receive clear, step-by-step instructions from the PCA manager for accomplishing duties,

3) To be instructed in methods that are organized logically and that are time and effort efficient, and to receive those instructions and other communications delivered in a clear, direct, assertive manner which is neither weakly passive nor abusively aggressive,

4) To be provided with equipment and supplies which are adequate for performing assigned duties,

5) To perform duties in a pleasant and sanitary working environment which has an efficient physical layout,

6) To refuse to perform certain proposed duties for sufficient reason and with reasonable advance notice,

7) To receive from you the confidentiality, respect, and dignity as a human who has personal thoughts, values,

beliefs, relationships, activities, and a personal life in addition to providing PCA assistance,

8) To receive both appreciation and a monetary salary which are commensurate with the extent and quality of duties performed,

9) To make genuine mistakes, have certain inabilities, and have limits to personal stamina, and

10) To resign with appropriate advance notice.

2. Two Approaches to "Aide/Attendant Instruction & Manuals"

There have been traditionally two approaches to providing details on the topic of "aide or attendant instruction":

a) Training the <u>aides</u> for those who will receive assistance, and

b) Training <u>those who require assistance</u> to be able to independently train & manage the aides whom they use.

a) Training <u>aides</u> for those who will receive assistance is essential for those service recipients who are either unable or unwilling to manage their own assistance. For others who are capable of managing the help which they use, a "pre-trained aide" can be a convenience but usually not a necessity. In either situation however, most circumstances additionally require that the recipient of services, or their representative, have sufficient skills to further initially instruct and manage the final, fine details of an individual's particular needs on a daily basis.

> Even aides with extensive training & experience will usually need instruction and daily management from each individual whom they assist

Regardless of either how extensive or formal a program is in attempting to train aides, it cannot instruct each aide in the specific needs which each individual will have for assistance. Most recipients -- or their personal representatives, when the individual is unable to state his own needs -- will be required to further train the aide in the details of their own specific needs for assistance. Whether an aide is a formally certified home health aide, or has instead received merely a workshop briefing on the type of work involved, that assistant will be usually making one key request on meeting each service recipient for the first time, "Please tell me what particular needs for assistance you have, and how and on what schedule you want me to provide that help."

Two Approaches to "Aide/Attendant Instruction & Manuals"   33

In addition to providing these initial instructions and training, the recipient must learn certain skills for the ongoing management of the help he receives. While an aide can be employed and somewhat supervised by an agency, the on-site management by the actual recipient of assistance is essential for maintaining a smooth relationship.

Therefore, those involved with home health aide or attendant training programs -- the administrators, instructors, nursing supervisors, aide/attendant trainees, and even the eventual recipients of services -- should guard against any assumption that "the aide training program will teach everything that the aide will forever need to know." Instead, as we have seen, the program primarily serves as an introduction or even a good foundation to the final instruction of specific details and on-site management which must take place between the aide and each recipient of services.

Regardless then, of whether aides are formally trained and supervised from a professional agency or merely briefed from an informal program, the services recipient or his representative must have certain skills for the daily, on-site management which even the best of agency supervisors cannot be constantly on-site to provide.

b) Training <u>those who use assistance</u>, or their representatives, to manage assistance provides them with essential management skills, while also promoting personal independence.

For service recipients who are able and willing to directly or indirectly manage their personal needs for assistance, a program which teaches one to independently manage that attendant assistance is far more important than a program which attempts to train aides or attendants for them. If only one program can be implemented, the program which trains capable recipients is essential, while the aide training program is sometimes a convenience but unnecessary.

The skills of managing one's own aide assistance is essential, whether one uses formally certified home health aides or college students who have no previous experience as attendants. We have illustrated in the previous section how important personal management skills are to instructing even highly trained aides in meeting the personal details of individual needs. In contrast to using certified aides, many folks who need assistance regularly recruit, interview and screen, train, and otherwise manage assistants who are willing to work but who have absolutely no related previous experience.

> The personal ability to recruit, train, & manage PCAs without agency help is becoming more and more important with today's shrinking supply of agency-employed aides

In using either type of assistance, clearly the personal ability to manage and instruct is essential.

This personal knowledge of managing assistance is also a major factor in the success of living independently. The reality of "independent living" is fully achievable even by those with disabilities which are sufficiently severe to require physical assistance from others...providing they can independently train and manage that assistance. Independent living is very difficult, if not impossible, when one is not in control of one's own daily schedule -- the ability to freely attend educational, career, and leisure activities -- or indeed, to at least maintain a basic quality of health in one's own living environment.

The skills of managing one's own attendant assistance gives one a maximum control over these factors. And the mere feeling of being in control plays a major factor in contributing to the feelings of assertiveness and self-esteem which are essential to successfully living independently.

Just a few years ago, neither a text nor a course existed which taught these management skills to the individual who actually uses assistance. One of the first texts, "Attendants and Attendees: A Guidebook of Helpful Hints," was published in two, 2,500-copy printings in 1979. Both printings were quickly exhausted in national distribution.

Two Approaches to "Aide/Attendant Instruction & Manuals"

The text of this book, by the same author, is an extensive revision of that much-requested 1979 version.

3. Why Should You Learn to Manage the Help You Use?

Consider 6 closely related "freedoms" which are yours when you learn to manage the assistance you use:

(1) Freedom to directly control the type, quality, and schedule of attendants -- and to change attendants -- whenever necessary

(2) Freedom from being dependent upon aide pools or referral agency lists, and the consequent ability to geographically relocate wherever and whenever necessary

(3) Freedom from having to use agency or college campus aide/attendant training services

(4) Freedom from having to pay the high hourly administrative rates to professional home health aide agencies, if one is not eligible for 3rd party funding

(5) Freedom from having to use parents or relatives as attendants

(6) Freedom from having to use a spouse, lover, or friend as an aide, or sole aide

> Management skills give you the freedom of a more independent lifestyle, & the ability to relieve loved ones of attendant responsibilities

Let's explore each of these six freedoms in detail:

(1) Freedom to directly control the type, quality, and schedule of attendants -- and to change attendants -- whenever necessary

If you personally owned a fancy restaurant which had a very posh reputation and your restaurant employed waiters, you -- as the owner -- would certainly want direct control over hiring those waiters. You would make sure that each waiter who worked in your restaurant was efficient, punctual, dependable, neat and clean in appearance, respectful in

Why Should You Learn to Manage the Help You Use? 37

greeting your public, and either already knowledgeable or willing to learn about being the best waiter possible.

Clearly, you would want control over the type, quality, and schedules of your waiters. You would not tolerate being told that someone else would hire all of your waiters for you, that you would be forced to use whatever waiters were referred to you by an employment service, that you would have to open and close your restaurant each day merely according to whenever waiters from the service happened to show up for work, or (heavens!) that you would have to share the same waiters with 3 other restaurants!

If a restaurant owner would insist on direct control over waiters who serve other people, then why should people who require assistance for personal needs settle for anything less?

Yet many attendant referral programs found at home health agencies, college campuses, and independent living centers do manage personal care attendants _for_ individuals who need assistance in this way. Many programs recruit, screen, interview, attempt to train, and even supervise the salaries of attendants, instead of helping people who require assistance to acquire these skills for their own management and direct control.

Of course some people are either unable or unwilling to directly instruct and manage the help which they use. For them, the use of an agency or attendant coordination program to instruct and manage is essential. However, for others who are capable of managing, there is little reason not to learn management skills, and therefore be free from the limitations which come with using many coordinating services.

Even with the best coordinating services, when people who require assistance are assigned aides, manytimes they are quite limited in the type and quality of aides which they are given to use each day. In addition, many folks find that they must start and end their daily personal activities not according to their own schedule, but according to when their assigned aide shows up. In many instances, the agency schedules the same aide among several service recipients each day. If one of these "clients" on an attendant's morning list takes a bit longer to help than expected, or if the attendant is late getting to even the first morning client, then the attendant's arrival at every subsequent client is often delayed and each individual's personal schedule is affected unexpectedly. The preventative measure taken by some agencies against these delays from occurring is to strictly limit the amount of time that an aide can spend with a client to the exact amount of scheduled time; consequently, any unexpected "accidents" or other personal needs of a client simply cannot be accommodated!

The answer to avoiding these problems, for those capable of managing the assistance they use, is to take a bit of time to learn how to take direct control over hiring and firing of the aides who are personally used...direct control over their type, quality, and schedule. Management skills make it possible to control these factors and to change attendants whenever necessary.

(2) Freedom from being dependent upon aide pools or referral agency lists, and the consequent ability to geographically relocate wherever and whenever necessary

Many agency services maintain a pool or listing of people who are willing to provide aide help. An aide pool can be quite helpful to an individual who has either just moved into a new geographical area or who has not yet developed skills for recruiting aides on their own. First, the newcomer usually needs aide help immediately upon arrival to the new area, before (it would seem) one's own recruiting could take place. Second, the newcomer may not be familiar right away with resources for personally recruiting aides in the new city or college campus.

While a home health aide agency or an attendant pool is helpful to many such newcomers, it is not essential. As we shall see later in this book, very competent attendants can be hired, sight unseen, from a thousand miles away. Surely, not every individual who requires assistance and who has moved to a new section of the country has either convinced an old attendant to move with them or chosen their new homestead only according to where there was another attendant pool!

Why Should You Learn to Manage the Help You Use? 39

Furthermore, we, as people who need assistance can become detrimentally dependent on a local, handy attendant pool. Even after becoming well established at a community or college campus, we naturally find that using the pool is sometimes easier than doing our own recruiting. Before long, we don't even bother to think of recruiting on our own, and we find that we are quite dependent on that pool. In fact, manytimes an individual never even bothers to learn how to recruit, because they have become so comfortably dependent on using the pool as their only means to finding new attendants.

This dependence -- like any other type -- can lead to your losing control of your life and to limiting your personal freedom and independence.

Now if attendant pools used by referral agencies always met one's attendant needs adequately, or if they could exist everywhere, then there certainly would be no objection to becoming comfortably dependent upon them. But the truth is that there are many problems with the consistency in the existence of pools and listings. It is not uncommon for the aide or attendant pool used by an agency or service to have "dry spells" when a supply of aides is not constantly available due to the agency's recruiting problems. The service's inability to supply aides may be quite temporary or prolonged in duration. The inability may mean that if this morning's aide is unable to work, several hours might elapse before a replacement can be recruited by the agency...or the delay might last several days.

> Using aides from agencies is essential for some people, however even those people will still require a certain level of skills for managing the aides and providing instruction on personal details

Furthermore, sooner or later, almost everyone finds the need to move away from the local pool of an agency, campus, or independent living center. As we have shown by exploring the other freedoms, being able to manage one's own attendant help enables one maximum flexibility to relocate residence locales wherever and whenever necessary. Geograpically relocating where one lives is almost as certain to happen these days as "death and taxes." If you know how to recruit and manage your own attendant help, you certainly have greater freedom of where and when you can move, as you will be able to recruit and hire your own attendants almost anywhere you go.

Yes, sooner or later, if you use aide or attendant help, you will find that it is wise to take a little time to learn how to recruit that help and maintain a personal list of replacements with your own resources. It really isn't that difficult.

(3) Freedom from having to use agency or college campus aide/attendant training services

In addition to maintaining attendant pools, many professional agencies, college campuses, and independent living centers provide attendant training services. These programs usually attempt to train attendants _for_ individuals who require assistance. The actual services vary, but they can include recruiting, interviewing, screening, conveying an awareness of the appropriate role of an attendant, training in the delivery of a wide variety of personal care services, assigning an attendant to an individual (or the same one to several individuals), and possibly even supervising an attendant's time sheets and salary payments.

An attendant training program which performs all or part of these functions can be a benefit to someone who hasn't yet learned how to be independent in managing that help. Pretrained aides are also essential to those who are unable or unwilling to train and manage assistance, themselves. However for those capable of managing, an attendant training program, like a constantly available attendant pool, has the potential to detrimentally postpone one's eventual need to personally learn these management skills. The individual who begins to rely on these services too many times doesn't bother to learn how to independently perform these procedures. Consequently, when she inevitably moves from this locale, she is finally faced with the need to suddenly learn the attendant management procedures which have been performed for her by the training program.

Ironically, the individual would already have developed the self-sufficient skills if the "helpful" attendant training program had not existed!

In addition, regardless of how poorly or how well a training program works, people who need assistance must inevitably provide the final details of instruction to each aide about our own particular needs. A program usually teaches a group of prospective aides in the generic types of help which they might be asked to deliver, since the program cannot predict the specific needs of each individual whom each attendant will be helping, and therefore which specific services each attendant should learn. When one who needs assistance initially meets even the best trained, most experienced aide, that aide is certain to make the key request, "Please instruct me as to what specific needs you have and the manner and schedule in which you would prefer your particular duties performed."

Consequently, a college campus or independent living center program which is truly interested in helping people prepare for self-sufficient, independent living should offer first a well structured program to train those who use assistance, and possibly second a program to train those who provide assistance.

Sooner or later, if you use attendant help, you should take a bit of time and learn how to manage the help which you use without the need to rely on a formal attendant training service to manage and train aides for you.

(4) Freedom from having to pay the high hourly administrative rates to professional home health aide agencies, if one is not eligible for 3rd party funding

A primary professional source for finding aides or attendants in many communities is a home health aide agency. The agency recruits, trains, schedules, pays, and otherwise manages aides for you. These services are very important to many folks, especially to those who are new to a locale and unsure where to find aides on their own, those with brief impairments or illnesses, those for whom aide services are funded and the funding source requires the use of agency-supplied aides, and to those who are unable or unwilling to manage their own attendant assistance.

There are several "prices" which one pays in return for these services. As we have discussed in previous "freedoms," you will realize some inflexibility in not being able to quickly change your personal schedule once an aide on a set schedule has been assigned. You will also lack the full freedom of changing aides from those assigned to you if problems occur. In addition, you may find that a replacement aide is not readily available from the agency's pool in case your regular aide doesn't arrive as scheduled.

Furthermore, the agency aides who help you manytimes are restricted by the agency in the amount of time which they can spend with you, which is unfortunate if unpredictable "accidents" happen. In addition, agencies often restrict aides in the types of work they can perform for you, as contrasted with the numerous types of work which you can request your own attendants to perform.

A further price is the monetary one. The agency charges administrative fees for its management services as well as other overhead expenses, in addition to the hourly salary which it actually pays the home health aides employed for you. The total of these agency fees often range from at least 25% in addition to the aide's actual hourly salary to as much as three or four times the aide's salary. For example, if an aide is paid $6 an hour, the total fee charged by the professional agency could range from $7.50 to over $25 per hour of provided assistance. Agencies are paid primarily by wealthy 3rd party funding sources, such as governmental departments and insurance companies. Many gainfully employed, private citizens are not eligible for long term, 3rd party funding and cannot afford agency rates on their own.

As mentioned, home health aide agencies do provide an important function to folks who need them. However, if you are able to manage your own attendant assistance, or you cannot afford the agency fees from your own pocket, you will be wise to learn management skills in order to substitute for costly agency services.

(5) Freedom from having to use parents or relatives as attendants

Many people with disabilities currently reside with attendant help which is provided entirely by parents or relatives. For some, this is a very satisfactory living situation. For others, there is a wish either to continue to live with one's folks but to supplement the attendant help they provide with some outside help, or to actually move out of the household to the independence of a new location across the neighborhood or across the country.

There are many justifiable reasons for wishing to relocate. They include the desire to pursue career training at a college, university, or vocational school, or to pursue a career, itself. Other folks who require assistance simply yearn for the privacy and independence of living on their own...or maybe they have their sights set on a potential lover or spouse!

Perhaps you would like to relocate on your own, but hesitate to do so because you are unsure of whether you could find help which is as reliable as that which your parents currently provide. Or maybe you are confident that you could find other help, but your parents lack that same confidence and pressure you to consequently stay home.

> Use help from hired PCAs for certain times when your relative, lover, or spouse needs a break; however, use help from those close to you for more private times

Regardless of the reason, we as people who need assistance must recognize that there will most definitely come a time in the future when our parents or relatives will no longer be able to provide us with attendant help. Our parents will either become of an age when they will no longer be physically able to help, or our brothers and sisters will someday be moving out to their own homestead.

Attendant help from the outside world can, indeed, be just as reliable as that which our parents and relatives provide. There will most certainly come a day when each one of us will need to know how to manage that outside help, and it is wise to begin preparing now, in advance of that potentially sudden need.

(6) Freedom from having to use a spouse, lover, or friend as an aide, or sole aide

Whether you have a lover or spouse, or you are hoping to find one, both of you should know that there are alternatives to having your mate automatically assume all of your attendant needs.

You and your spouse or lover understandably want as much privacy as possible. Manytimes the first inclination for a new couple is to do away with outside attendants. The mate therefore begins to assume all attendant responsibilities, perhaps a total amount of help which had been formerly divided each day -- or should have been divided -- among two or more aides...and with good reason.

Perhaps your needs were divided because they were too extensive for one attendant to handle 7 days a week, week after week, month after month. As we shall see later in this book, if daily needs for attendant help are extensive, they should be divided among two or more attendants to avoid unnecessarily fatiguing a single attendant. This unnecessary fatigue can result in a frequent turnover of overworked attendants quitting...something which you should prevent from happening to a mate whom you wish to keep for lifetime. In addition, you should not be dependent only on help from your mate in case she becomes sick or injured and suddenly is not able to help you for an undeterminable period of time.

Remember, a decision to hire outside help for at least some daily needs is not a sign of your lover rejecting you or of an unstable romantic relationship. On the contrary, it is a step toward avoiding these problems from happening!

The answer to avoiding unnecessary fatigue for your mate is to delegate at least some of your attendant needs to outside help. Careful choice should be made when deciding which attendant needs will be assigned to outside help. A high priority might be given to certain duties, possibly because of

Why Should You Learn to Manage the Help You Use?   45

their heavy physical nature (such as lifting) or their routine occurrence at a time when your mate would like to be doing something else (such as a hobby, a career, or merely taking "time out"). On the other hand, outside help should not be used for times which would interrupt certain private activities which you and your mate value. Examples include certain romantic mornings when you both can sleep late, or certain intimate evenings when both of you can routinely stay up late!

In summary, we have discussed six significant freedoms which you can enjoy by taking the time to learn management skills. These freedoms have addressed putting you in control of the assistance that you require, and preventing some needless problems from occurring.

4. The 3 Management Situations: Which One Applies to You?

If you have valid needs for physical assistance from PCAs, you will probably find your personal situation described in one of the 3 management situations illustrated in this section. These 3 situations describe 3 categories of ability and desire to manage.

It is important to realize which situation describes your circumstance so that you, or those who represent you, will better know how to use the management skills in this book. And yes, you can still manage the people who assist you even if physical, visual, or verbal limitations prevent you from independently performing all of the management and supervisory duties...read on.

Before these 3 management situations are described in detail, each will be graphically presented. After these graphics, the detailed descriptions will begin with one set of universal comments which apply to all 3 management situations. After the universal comments, each of the 3 situations will be described separately.

Situation One

> You Have the Personal Desire and the Psychological, Physical, Visual, Auditory, and Verbal Abilities to Manage PCAs

Step One. The Sources of Medical Details (initial & ongoing)

> Physicians, Nurses, Therapists,& Other Health Professionals

Step Two. The Receiver of Medical Details

> You, as Both the Manager & Recipient of PCA Services

Step Three. The Providers of Physical Assistance

> PCAs Who Assist You

Situation Two

> You Have The Personal Desire and the Psychological Ability to Manage PCAs, But are Hampered by the Inability to Physically Manage PCAs, Meet Visual Requirements of Some Paperwork, or to Audibly or Verbally Communicate

Step One. The Sources of Medical Details (initial & ongoing)

> Physicians, Nurses, Therapists, & Other Health Professionals

Step Two. The Receiver of Medical Details

> You, as Both the Manager & Recipient of PCA Services

Step Three. The Coordinator of Assistance Providers

> The PCA Coordinator (can be of medical or non-medical background) You directly manage the PCA Coordinator who, in turn, accommodates your inabilities by managing only those physical, visual, or verbal management tasks which you cannot perform.

Step Four. The Providers of Physical Assistance

> PCAs Who Assist You

Situation Three

> You Do Not Have the Personal Desire or the Psychological Ability to Manage PCAs

Step One. The Sources of Medical Details (initial & ongoing)

> Physicians, Nurses, Therapists, & Other Health Professionals

Step Two. The Receiver of Medical Details & The Manager of Assistance Providers

> The PCA Manager (family member, medical professional, or nursing/home health aide agency) The PCA Manager consults with medical professionals and you to determine your needs, and then manages the PCAs for you

Step Three. The Recipient of Physical Assistance

> You, as the Recipient of PCA Services

Step Four. The Providers of Physical Assistance

> PCAs Who Assist You

Universal Comments

Step One.
In the first step of each of the 3 management situations, the medical knowledge and management authority begins with the "physicians, nurses, therapists, and other health professionals."

These are the medical professionals of different disciplines from whom you have received different types of medical care in an institutional, clinical, or office setting, and probably as both an in-patient and out-patient at various times. These professionals were the first to know the details of your medical concerns and background, because they were the ones to diagnose and treat it. You first learned from them of your medical details, physical abilities and inabilities, and the consequent needs and medical methods for receiving physical help from others in order to accommodate your inabilities.

You should realize that these professionals will continue to be the main advisory resource on medical information. They can advise you or the Manager who acts on your behalf. Their advice should be requested whenever it is needed.

Step Two.
The second step in each situation is occupied by whoever communicates directly with the health professionals regarding details of your care. In the first two management situations you are in charge of management, and therefore you should be the direct recipient of medical details from the medical professionals in step one.

In fact, after just a short time of consulting with a number and variety of medical professionals on various issues, you should become a more knowledgeable reference about your total medical background than any single medical professional. You should eventually become the best historical record on your own medical diagnosis, treatments, abilities, inabilities, and warning signs which you have experienced and which herald upcoming medical problems.

This does not mean that you should refuse to seek help from medical professionals, but it does mean that you should become the most complete and instantly available layman's reference on your own history for professionals to tap as needed. This means developing a routine habit of asking sincere questions during treatments so that you understand a reasonable amount of detail, and then at least mentally store the answers which you receive.

Because of this unique expertise which you can develop on your own medical background, you will be the only one who needs to consult with "physicians, nurses, therapists, and other health professionals" in Situations One and Two. However, in Situation Three, if you lack the desire or psychological ability to know your own medical background, then the PCA Manager who acts on your behalf will be the one to review your needs with these medical professionals.

For further details on each of the 3 situations, please consult the flow charts and the expanded notes which follow.

Situation One

> You Have the Personal Desire and the Psychological, Physical, Visual, Auditory, and Verbal Abilities to Manage PCAs

Step One. The Sources of Medical Details (initial & ongoing)

> Physicians, Nurses, Therapists, & Other Health Professionals

Step Two. The Receiver of Medical Details

> You, as Both the Manager & Recipient of PCA Services

Step Three. The Providers of Physical Assistance

> PCAs Who Assist You

You are described in Situation One if you have the desire and the psychological ability to manage the PCA assistance which you require. In addition, you have the basic physical and visual ability to manage the assistance and the ability to verbally communicate readily with those assisting you.

With these abilities, you can be directly in charge of management if you wish to be...and as we will see in Situation Two, many people without these physical, visual, or verbal abilities still manage their own assistance!

Procedure for Managing in Situation One

From the beginning of your illness or impairment, you have been interested and involved with the diagnoses and treatments from the "physicians, nurses, therapists, and other health professionals" who have helped you. You have asked sincere questions from the onset of your condition regarding why it occurred, methods for routinely caring for the condition, symptoms of typical nonroutine problems, and commonsense remedies for nonroutine problems. In short, you have a good layman's understanding of your medical history, how to take care of yourself, and what to do when certain, minor problems occur.

In addition to this initial information, you have made a continuing habit of asking questions of health professionals who treat you. Consequently, you have become the best reference available to these health professionals regarding your medical history and, when a problem occurs, providing much of the information which professionals need in diagnosing and treating you.

As a result of your good relationship with health professionals, and your solid layman's knowledge of how to care for yourself, you are fully qualified to manage the physical assistance which you need from others. Once you learned how to care for yourself, you next learned and have habitually performed independently all of the details of care which you can physically perform for yourself.

Those details of your own care which you cannot physically perform for yourself, and for which you require assistance from others, are the duties for which you manage help from PCAs. Consequently, you directly manage the PCAs who assist you.

In Situation One, you are both the manager and the services recipient, and the PCAs who assist you look solely to you for instruction and managerial supervision.

Situation Two

> You Have The Personal Desire and the Psychological Ability to Manage PCAs, But are Hampered by the Inability to Physically Manage PCAs, Meet Visual Requirements of Some Paperwork, or to Audibly or Verbally Communicate

Step One. The Sources of Medical Details (initial & ongoing)

> Physicians, Nurses, Therapists, & Other Health Professionals

Step Two. The Receiver of Medical Details

> You, as Both the Manager & Recipient of PCA Services

Step Three. The Coordinator of Assistance Providers

> The PCA Coordinator (can be of medical or non-medical background) You directly manage the PCA Coordinator who, in turn, accommodates your inabilities by managing only those physical, visual, or verbal management tasks which you cannot perform.

Step Four. The Providers of Physical Assistance

> PCAs Who Assist You

You are described in Situation Two if you have the desire and the psychological ability to manage assistance, but you are hampered by a significant inability to physically manage assistance, to visually coordinate some of the paperwork, or to audibly or verbally communicate readily.

We are not assuming that such inabilities mean a total impediment to managing assistance or that a Coordinator is always necessary. Many, many folks with such physical, visual, audible, or verbal management impairments, or partial impairments, are still the sole managers of their

PCA assistance. If you have significant physical impairments in these areas, but are determined to not use a Coordinator, then by all means jump up into some modification of Situation One with our encouragement.

We have designed Situation Two, however, for those people who find that significant impairments do present significant difficulties in independently performing the physical points of management (the physical requirements of recruiting, screening applicants, filling out weekly PCA work schedules or salary forms, and the like), the visual requirements of some paperwork, or in hearing or verbally communicating complex instructions and supervision to someone as they assist you.

Procedure for Managing in Situation Two

Just as in Situation One, you have become fully knowledgeable about your medical history and the details of your own care.

From the beginning of your illness or impairment, you have been interested and involved with the diagnoses and treatments from the "physicians, nurses, therapists, and other health professionals" who have helped you. You have asked sincere questions from the onset of your condition regarding why it occurred, methods for routinely caring for the condition, symptoms of typical nonroutine problems, and commonsense remedies for nonroutine problems. In short, you have a good layman's understanding of your medical history, how to take care of yourself, and what to do when problems occur.

In addition to this initial information, you have made a continuing habit of asking questions of health professionals who treat you. Consequently, you have become the best reference available to these health professionals regarding your medical history and, when a problem occurs, providing much of the information which professionals need in diagnosing and treating you.

As a result of your good relationship with health professionals, and your solid layman's knowledge of how to care for yourself, you are fully qualified to manage the physical assistance which you need from others. Once you learned how to care for yourself, you next learned and have habitually performed independently all of the details of care which you can physically perform for yourself.

Those details of your own care which you cannot physically perform for yourself, and for which you require assistance from others, are the duties for which you manage help from PCAs.

In addition to not being able to physically perform all the details of your own care, you have determined that there are certain tasks involved in <u>managing</u> PCAs which you cannot physically, visually, or verbally perform.

If these are big management impediments to you, they should still not prevent you from being a manager-in-charge. You may wish to consider training and using a PCA Coordinator. With a Coordinator you are still in charge, because the Coordinator receives her instructions only from you. This is a process in managenment circles known as "delegating." After all, the chairmen of major corporations are fully in charge, eventhough they rarely perform all of the physical, visual, and verbal duties of management. That's why Lee Iaccoca has foremen, or coordinators, carrying out his instructions on the car assemblyline!

Since you are the manager as well as the expert reference on your own medical background and physical needs, you do not need someone with a medical expertise as your Coordinator...just as the PCAs whom you manage do not need medical expertise. You are the only necessary medical reference for Situations One and Two, however you should feel free to consult the advice of those "physicians, nurses, therapists, and other health professionals" whenever you have questions.

Your Coordinator, indeed, could be your most experienced PCA whom you have promoted to the Coordinator position with a slight increase in salary. In this case of a promotion, you will have very little training to do because your Coordinator, as a previous PCA, already knows your needs. Depending upon the number of duties which the Coordinator will be performing, she might spend all of her time coordinating, or she might be a part-time PCA and a part-time Coordinator.

Yes, you are the ultimate authority and manager, and it is just as important that the Coordinator and the PCAs understand and respect your position as it is for the car assemblyline workers to understand that their foreman is a coordinator, but that Lee Iaccoca is the true manager. It is also important that you understand your managerial responsibilities, and that you do not get lazy and delegate all management responsibilities to your Coordinator. The Coordinator should be used only for those specific physical, visual, or verbal details of management which you cannot independently perform...a kind of specialized PCA.

Situation Three

> You Do Not Have the Personal Desire or the Psychological Ability to Manage PCAs

Step One. The Sources of Medical Details (initial & ongoing)

> Physicians, Nurses, Therapists, & Other Health Professionals

Step Two. The Receiver of Medical Details & The Manager of Assistance Providers

> The PCA Manager (family member, medical professional, or nursing/home health aide agency) The PCA Manager consults with medical professionals and you to determine your needs, and then manages the PCAs for you

Step Three. The Recipient of Physical Assistance

> You, as the Recipient of PCA Services

Step Four. The Providers of Physical Assistance

> PCAs Who Assist You

You are described in Situation Three if you do not desire to manage your PCA assistance or if you lack the psychological ability to manage.

Many folks validly fall into Situation Three for either of two reasons. In one case, folks have the ability to manage, but simply choose not to do so, and are very passive about the care which they need as well as life in general. The second type, by no choice of their own, are truly unable to mentally or emotionally manage due to the nature of their illness, impairment, disability, progressive age, or other reasons.

The 3 Management Situations

Procedure for Managing in Situation Three

For either type of individual in Situation Three, there is usually some sort of lack of desire or inability to sufficiently know or remember one's medical background and personal needs, added to the inability to adequately solve problems, make decisions, and to otherwise manage the PCA assistance.

Regardless, one's requirement for physical assistance still exists and this need must be managed by someone. The PCA Manager assumes most or all of the responsibility for receiving medical details as well as the direct management and supervision of the PCAs.

Since the recipient of services in Situation Three is not knowledgeable about their own medical needs, the PCA Manager must have this knowledge. This means that the Manager can be a spouse or close family member who has simply learned the medical needs of the individual. An alternative is that the Manager can be a professional with medical expertise, such as those found in a home health aide agency or in a care institution such as a nursing home.

In Situation Three, the Manager consults both with the individual requiring assistance and with the "physicians, nurses, therapists, and other health professionals" who know the individual. Then they compile an inventory of medical background and physical needs, and proceed to train and manage the physical assistance for the individual.

The recipient of services in Situation Three is usually quite passive about the details and quality of the care they need. The Manager assumes these responsibilities.

Section II

Strategies for Being a Good Manager

5) The Top 10 Reasons Why PCAs Quit & Are Fired

6) Settings in Which You Use Help

7) Types of Help & the Services Which Each Provider Performs

8) Qualities and Strategies of a Good Manager

9) Passive, Aggressive, & Assertive: Which Style is Best for Stating Needs?

10) Job Expectations

11) The Favorable Physical Work Environment

5. The Top 10 Reasons Why PCAs Quit & Are Fired

As one of the first steps to learning the strategies of a good manager, it is important to review the primary reasons why PCA employees quit their undesirable jobs, from the PCA's point of view, as well as why unsatisfactory PCAs are fired from their jobs, from the employer's point of view.

In short, what we have here are the main traits which either make a PCA job or manager undesirable, or make a PCA employee unsatisfactory. These are closely related to many of the previously listed "Rights for You and the PCA."

The Top 10 Reasons Why PCAs Quit their Jobs

1) They receive an incomplete list of duties or procedural instructions on being hired, and they become frustrated as unexpected duties are sporadically and frequently added.

2) The methods and step-by-step order for performing duties are not logical and waste the time and effort of the PCA.

3) Their working environment is unpleasant and frustrating because it lacks adequate supplies or is disorganized, poorly layed out, dirty, strewn with garbage, piled with dirty laundry, and is dusty, dark, musty, smelly of urine or bowel, or infested with bugs or rodents.

> You can be a better manager by understanding the reasons why PCAs quit their jobs, as well as why they are most often fired

4) They are not paid a sufficient monetary salary, or given scheduled salary increases when expected or, in addition to monetary salaries, their supervisor fails to routinely express to them appropriate appreciation for their work.

5) When more than one PCA is employed the supervisor obviously favors one employee over another, tolerates one PCA routinely leaving unfinished duties for the next PCA to complete, speaks unfavorably to either PCA about the other,

or in similar ways tolerates or contributes to gossip, favoritism, unfair advantages, or injustices,

6) Their supervisor is not appropriately assertive, and instead is either weakly passive or abusively aggressive during daily communications and relations of expressing standard needs, special needs, changes in duties or schedule, opinions, preferences, and feelings,

7) Their supervisor is dishonest regarding their possessions, time worked, or salary owed, or has hidden expectations such as expecting sexual favors or loans of money or possessions,

8) Their supervisor is abusive, unreasonable, and stressful in demanding that duties be performed which are inappropriate because the supervisor could do them for himself, that duties be performed which are not appropriate for the PCA to perform, that duties be performed which are too numerous for a specific period of work time, that duties must be performed with unnecessary speed or urgency, or that duties be performed under unnecessarily tight supervision,

9) Their supervisor is intolerent of their honest mistakes of occasionally forgetting details, being unable to physically perform certain duties, or needing occasional sick or personal time from duties, and

10) Their supervisor fails to respect their personal lives, rights, time, or other concerns by assuming that the standard job responsibilities and schedules, as well as changes, should take priority over an employee's personal life.

The Top 10 Reasons Why PCAs are Fired from their Jobs

1) They are repeatedly undependable in arriving at all for work, they often attempt to arrive late or leave early, or they fail to call in advance to notify of upcoming inabilities to arrive on schedule,

2) They are not reasonably clean and professional in personal hygiene, clothing, language, or habits,

The Top 10 Reasons Why PCAs Quit & Are Fired

3) They jeopardize the safety or health of the individual whom they assist by performing a poor quality of work, not observing the safe procedural methods requested by their employer, becoming physically or verbally abusive, or working under the influence of drugs, medications, or alcohol,

4) They prove to be physically, psychologically, or emotionally unable to perform the duties, or unreasonably slow or lazy while working,

5) They are dishonest with their employer's work time, possessions, finances, medications, or food, or similarly dishonest with fellow PCA employees in routinely not completing assigned duties and purposely leaving them for completion by the PCA of the following work shift,

6) They lack respect for their employer's rights and his need for confidentiality and privacy with regard to preferences, opinions, feelings, problems, values, beliefs, relationships, and activities, and consequently they gossip and speak too freely to outsiders about their employer's private life,

7) They have an inappropriate attitude toward people with disabilities and lack respect for their employer as an individual who, regardless of physical sickness or impairments, has a mind which is fully capable of knowing personal needs, making decisions, and managing the physical assistance which their body requires,

8) They try to take control of their employer's right to make decisions regarding the selection and number of employed PCAs, the choice of specific duties to be performed, the procedural methods and schedule for those duties, and the quality and dependability of assistance which is required,

9) They are not appropriately assertive, and instead are either weakly passive or abusively aggressive during daily communications and relations of expressing standard needs, special needs, changes in duties or schedule, opinions, preferences, and feelings, and

10) They simply do not want to continue to perform the duties of the work according to the schedule, methods, and

amount of salary which their employer requires and to which they originally agreed.

6. Settings in Which You Use Help

Very few of us spend our entire lives solely within the interior walls of our living area. We use our living area as a home base from which we travel to take part in a variety of daily activities throughout the surrounding community and beyond. We leave our home base during the day or evening to reach appointments and meetings, social and leisure activities, and in order to meet educational or career responsibilities on a punctual, routine schedule. Many of us enjoy overnight stays during vacation or business trips. Occasionally, it may also be necessary to stay in a hospital or rehabilitation center if short term ailments or new impairments occur.

If we are physically dependent on others for certain routine needs, we will probably have a degree of dependence for assistance in whatever activity we choose. It is important to realize that physical assistance is usually available in almost any setting, for almost any type of activity, and that we should not limit our activity planning to whatever can occur within the walls of our home base.

This section shows where to find and how to properly use PCA help in 8 different activity settings. You should not feel limited to the brief information provided here in planning what types of activities are possible or where to find assistance which you might require.

Setting: Acute Care Hospital

Purpose
Short term medical care and therapies with the objective of curing some ailments or minimizing the negative effects of others; possible referral for further care to a rehabilitation hospital, nursing home, or care at home

Typical Contacts for Care or Assistance
Physician, nurse, aide, therapist, & other health professionals

Titles of Your Relationship to Those Who Provide Assistance
1) Patient, for medical care to your nonroutine ailment

2) Manager, for assistance required for your routine personal needs

Your Role in These Relationships
1) As a patient, to provide medical professionals with details about your current symptoms of illness as well as about your medical history, to receive and discuss the physician's diagnosis and treatment plan, to learn about your ailment and participate in decisions, to participate in your medical care and therapies while monitoring their quality, to learn your responsibilities for post-discharge self-care, and to consult with health professionals after discharge whenever necessary

2) As a manager, to inform staff contacts of the equipment, procedures, & schedules that you routinely follow in your needs for physical assistance from others; to be willing to compromise on equipment types, procedures, & schedules around those available in the hospital, but not to compromise on the quality of assistance which you receive

Once in a while, each of us encounters a new ailment or an additional impairment which necessitates in-patient care at an acute care hospital.

The objective for this care is curing some types of ailments or reducing the negative effects of other ailments when a complete cure is not possible. The end result of the hospital stay might be a restriction-free discharge to one's previous living environment, or a referral for further care or therapies to a rehabilitation hospital or center, nursing home, or care at home.

The typical, most common contacts during a hospital stay include a physician, nurse, aide, therapists, and other health professionals. The titles of your relationship with these professionals are primarily 2-fold as both a patient and a manager.

Your status as a patient applies while you receive medical care and therapies for an ailment which is not part of your normal routine. As a patient, you should feel free to ask questions and to monitor and participate in the care you receive, but you primarily entrust your ailment to the wisdom of medical professionals and follow their suggestions and instructions. Further responsibilities of a patient include learning at least the basics about your ailment to enable observing, monitoring, and participating in the medical care. In addition, it is important to learn about your own personal responsibilities for your care after discharge, and to realize that you are welcome to call or consult with these professionals at anytime in the future when you need medical advice.

The hospital stay is a mixture of patient care for a nonroutine ailment as well as the usual requirements for physical assistance for your routine needs. For those routine needs, such as grooming, bathing, eating, and toileting, you should change roles from being a hospital patient who follows suggestions and instructions to being a manager of assistance who politely and assertively makes your needs known and provides instruction on how to assist those needs. For these routine needs, the nurse or aide will typically state, "If you would like any assistance with such-and-such activity, please feel free to let me know what kind of help you need and how I can best provide it."

As your own manager, you should make your needs known with regard to the equipment, procedures, and schedule or logical order which you usually follow. It is wise to discuss these factors early, perhaps at the admissions check-in when you first arrive in your room, with the primary nurse assigned to you. The primary nurse will ask you standard admission questions about your health, medical condition, usual diet, and the medications which you normally take. This is an ideal, early time to discuss the types of physical assistance you will need as well as how long you typically require assistance with each activity. If you require 45 minutes of assistance in the morning with a bed bath, your primary nurse should know this in advance to enable staff planning. Be prepared to make reasonable compromises about the types of equipment, procedures, and schedules around those which are available in this temporary, hospital setting. Think of your stay as an adventure challenge or game of "camping out" for a few days where you will not have all of the comforts or schedule of home.

Do not compromise, however, on the overall quality of care or assistance which you receive; do not "do without" routine needs just because the nurse seems too busy to help you or the aide yelled at you. If you encounter problems, try to explain the reasons why some part of your routine care is important to you and see if the reaction of the nurse or aide changes. If problems cannot be resolved in this way, ask to speak with your primary nurse or the nursing supervisor. Explain the problem as objectively as you can, with a minimum of emotions or any trace of arrogant aggressiveness, and ask for the nurse's advice in resolving the matter. Again, further compromises in methods -- but not quality -- might be necessary. For tips on appropriate ways of communicating, see chapter 9, "Passive, Aggressive, and Assertive."

Feel free to refer to the "Patient's Bill of Rights" which you probably received from the hospital at the admissions check-in. Almost every hospital issues such a listing to new patients. Refer to this listing if you wish specifics about your individual rights in the hospital, or if you simply wish some reassurance and confidence that the topic about which you are about to complain is justified. For your convenient reference, a typical listing is provided below.

Patient's Bill of Rights

As a Patient at Boston General Hospital, You Shall Have The Right To:

1) Receive emergency medical treatment as indicated by your medical condition upon arrival to the Emergency Department.

2) Considerate and respectful care.

3) The name of the physician responsible for coordinating your care.

4) The name and function of any person providing health care services to you.

5) Obtain from your physician complete current information concerning your diagnosis, treatment, and prognosis in terms you can reasonably be expected to understand. When it is not medically advisable to give you such information, this information shall be available to an appropriate person on your behalf.

6) Receive from your physician information necessary to give informed consent prior to the start of any procedure, treatment, or both. This information, except for emergency situations not requiring an informed consent, shall include as a minimum the specific procedure or treatment or both, the medically significant risks involved, and the probable duration of incapacitation, if any. You will be advised of medically significant alternatives for care or treatment, if any.

7) Refuse treatment to the extent permitted by law and to be informed of the medical consequences of this action.

8) Privacy to the extent consistent with providing you adequate medical care. This shall not preclude discreet discussion of your case or examination of you by appropriate medical personnel.

9) Privacy and confidentiality of all records pertaining to your treatment, except as otherwise provided by law or third party payment contract.

10) A response by the hospital to requests for usual services consistent with your treatment.

11) Be informed by your physician, or his designee, of your continuing health care requirements following discharge.

12) Receive information about the need to transfer you to another facility and any alternatives there might be to such a transfer.

13) The identity, upon request, of other health care and educational institutions that the hospital has authorized to participate in your treatment.

14) Refuse to participate in research and that human experimentation affecting your care and treatment; such shall be performed only with your informed consent.

15) Examine and receive an explanation of your bill, regardless of source of payment.

16) Treatment without discrimination as to race, color, religion, sex, national origin, handicap, or source of payment.

17) Designate any accommodation to which you are admitted as a nonsmoking area.

18) Without fear of reprisal, voice grievances and recommend changes in policies and services to our staff, the governing authority, and the New York State Department of Health.

19) Submit complaints about the hospital care and services and to have the hospital investigate such complaints. The hospital is responsible for providing you, if requested, with a written response indicating the findings of the investigation. If you are dissatisfied, the hospital will then direct you to the appropriate office of the Massachusetts Department of Health.

20) Know the hospital rules and regulations that apply to your conduct as a patient.

21) Free copies of the "Boston Globe," "Boston Herald," "Wall Street Journal," and "B.A.D. Phoenix" delivered to your room each day.

Setting: Rehabilitation Hospital

Purpose
Short term medical care and therapies with objectives of emotional adjustment & physical accommodation to a new lifestyle due to a disability

Typical Contacts for Care or Assistance
Physician, nurse, aide, therapist, & other health professionals

Titles of Your Relationship to Those Who Provide Assistance
1) Patient, for medical care to your nonroutine ailment

2) Student, in learning to emotionally adjust & physically accommodate to a new lifestyle resulting from a disability or impairment

3) Manager, for assistance required for those routine personal needs with which you are already familiar; become a manager in new areas of routine care as soon as you learn the methods

Your Role in These Relationships
1) As a patient, to provide medical professionals with details about your current symptoms of illness as well as about your medical history, to receive and discuss the physician's diagnosis and treatment plan, to learn about your ailment and participate in decisions, to participate in your medical care and therapies while monitoring their quality, to learn your responsibilities for post-discharge self-care, and to consult with health professionals after discharge whenever necessary

2) As a student, to learn and practice the emotional coping strategies and the physical accommodations as offered by physician, nurse, therapist, social worker/counselor, & other professionals

3) As a manager, to inform staff contacts of the equipment, procedures, & schedules that you routinely follow in your needs for physical assistance from others; to be willing to compromise on equipment types, procedures, & schedules around those available in the

Settings in Which You Use Help 75

hospital, but not to compromise on the quality of assistance which you receive

Occasionally, we find that a stay in a rehabilitation hospital or center is necessary in order to address a new impairment which has occurred or to re-evaluate an impairment which has existed for sometime.

The objective for the stay can include emotional adjustment or physical accommodation to a new or improved lifestyle which is due to an impairment, disability, or handicap. The typical contacts during the stay include the same kinds of medical professionals which were discussed for the acute care hospital. Your titles and roles toward these professionals include the same patient and manager functions as explained for a hospital stay, however in a rehabilitation hospital you have the additional title and role of a student.

As a student during your stay, you are wise to absorb all that you can of the education, information, strategies, and techniques which are offered during your stay by the various types of professionals around you. Some rehab patients are strongly tempted to discharge themselves early as a way to seemingly escape from their own impairment and the therapies and other rehab responsibilities which they must assume because of their own impairment. Some others become defensive against and reject the suggestions of professionals such as doctors, nurses, aides, physical therapists, occupational therapists, speech therapists, and counselors.

Instead of fighting them, think of these folks as your "presidential cabinet of advisors" who will be suggesting "short cuts" and "inside tips" on ways to get the most activity and enjoyment out of your life despite your impairment.

Be a willing, eager student in learning rehab techniques. Learn all that you can about your disability and ways to make the emotional adjustment as well as physical accommodations. In addition, ask advice in deciding between those activities which you can independently perform for yourself and those with which you realistically require physical assistance from others.

For the first category of activities, learn the short-cuts and tricks for doing all that you can for yourself. For the latter category, learn from the professionals around you about the most safe and efficient methods for performing the tasks so that you can clearly direct the physical assistance which you obtain from others...and begin managing that assistance as soon as possible.

Setting: Transitional & Residential Independent Living Center

Purpose
Short term, temporary residence where independent living skills are taught to enable the client an increased independence in a later institutional setting or in one's own private setting

Typical Contacts for Care and Assistance
Aide (from a home health aide agency or personal recruiting), skills instructor, & social worker, with visiting nurse & other health & vocational professionals on-call

Titles of Your Relationship to Those Who Provide Assistance
1) Student, in learning to emotionally adjust & physically accommodate to a new lifestyle resulting from a disability or impairment

2) Manager, for assistance required for those routine personal needs with which you are already familiar; become a manager in new areas of routine care as soon as you learn the methods

Your Role in These Relationships
1) As a student, to learn and practice the emotional coping strategies and the physical accommodations as offered by physician, nurse, therapist, social worker/counselor, & other professionals

2) As a manager, to inform staff contacts of the equipment, procedures, & schedules that you routinely follow in your needs for physical assistance from others; to be willing to compromise on equipment types, procedures, & schedules around those available in the hospital, but not to compromise on the quality of assistance which you receive

Before someone attempts to take advantage of an independent living program, they should have taken maximum advantage of the rehabilitation hospital resources since each of these two facilities has a separate area of expertise with very little overlap or duplication. For anyone who wishes advice on increasing their independent living skills beyond the resources offered at a rehabilitation hospital, there are two primary types of independent living programs or centers.

The most numerous type of independent living programs are non-residential programs which consist of a central office and a demonstration/classrooms area in which a variety of specialized counselors are headquartered. These counselors are available to individuals who either are able to visit the area in order to receive counseling, or who ask that a counselor comes to their home. In either case, the counselor can coach the individual on methods and strategies for increasing their independence in performing specific types of daily living activities.

In addition to independent living programs which are headquartered in this type of area, there is an increasing number of transitional and residential independent living centers. For admission to this type of program, the individual submits an application which details very firm reasons and personal goals for wishing to live at the residential center for a temporary period in order to learn skills. A progressive program will be very clear in stating that it has no room or time for housing residents who desire to be dependent, passive patients.

If accepted by the residential program, the individual lives in his assigned, private apartment within or nearby the center for a period of time which typically ranges from 6 to 18 months. During this time, each resident is expected to regularly participate in 2 primary types of skills training activities: individual counseling sessions about personal concerns and individual accommodation needs, and group classes and workshops which address concerns shared in common by most of the residents. Individual counseling might address ways of independently performing personal medical procedures and coping with specific problems of emotional adjustment. The group session topics might include PCA management skills, managing personal finances, assertiveness training, and others aimed at preparing for educational and career opportunities.

The overall purpose of a transitional and residential program is to teach independent living skills in a

Settings in Which You Use Help

residential setting where residents can feel free to make mistakes while counseling support is available. One is not always free to experiment with new independent living strategies while living in a protective home with parents or relatives or in a nursing home setting. The clear objective of the program is for each resident to make steady progress toward independently managing their own living needs, and then to move into a more independent setting which is appropriate to their abilities...hence, the reason the program is termed "transitional and residential."

Since the setting is designed to simulate living on one's own while the program provides professional support, the professional contacts differ from the previously discussed hospitals. Aides are available for the residents to share and directly manage themselves; skills instructors and counselors provide instruction and support; and nurses, therapists, and physicians are on-call for approach by residents, just as they will be during a future life in the community.

The titles of the resident's relationship to these professionals include "student," with the objective of learning independent living skills, and "manager," with the objective of learning and improving life management skills. These titles and roles have already been discussed in more detail for the two previous hospital settings.

Setting: Nursing Home or Infirmary

Purpose
Long term medical care and therapies with the objective of the institution managing and providing most needs for the dependent patient

Typical Contacts for Care and Assistance
Nurse, aide, and therapist with other health professionals usually on-call

Titles of Your Relationship to Those Who Provide Assistance
1) Patient, for medical care and assistance in areas where you do not have the ability or desire to manage

2) Manager, in those areas of routine personal needs where you have the ability and desire to manage

Your Role in These Relationships
1) If you are unable or choose not to manage as many of your personal needs as possible, then you become a patient who is totally dependent on decisions made by the staff about your needs and daily schedule.

2) As a manager, your desire to manage the assistance you require for certain personal needs might be met with some resistance by some staff who do not frequently encounter capable, assertive residents. In this event, an ongoing series of discussions with nursing home administrators may be necessary.

Nursing homes and infirmaries provide primarily long term medical care and therapies to those who are often unable or unwilling to manage significant portions of their personal needs.

The most common professional contacts at a nursing home include social workers, nurses, aides, and therapists, while physicians and other health professionals are usually available on an on-call basis.

The titles of the resident's relationship to these professionals are usually a mixture of "patient," for the majority of daily activities, and "manager," for a minority of activities. Residents usually become increasingly passive and dependent upon staff care and, as their stay continues, upon staff decisions. The price of being dependent on this care includes living by staff decisions with regard to their choice and schedule of daily activities. For many residents who become truly passive and dependent due to a mental inability to manage their own needs, this surrender of one's choices to decisions made by staff might not present significant problems. However, for those who are clear-thinking and consequently have the ability to manage but choose not to do so, the surrender of choices can cause an emotionally devastating and progressive depression.

Setting: Private Housing
   (House, Condo, Apartment, Etc.)

   Purpose
   Short or long term residence in one's own private setting

   Typical Contacts for Care and Assistance
   Relative, spouse, aide (from a home health agency or personal recruiting), or friend, with consultation access to a physician, visiting nurse, & other health professionals

   Titles of Your Relationship to Those Who Provide Assistance
   1) Patient, for medical care to nonroutine ailments, and for physical assistance to routine needs in areas where you do not have the ability or desire to manage

   2) Manager, in those areas of your routine personal needs where you have the ability and desire to manage

   Your Role in This Relationship
   1) If you are unable to manage or choose not to manage as many of your personal needs as possible, then you become a patient who is totally dependent on others around you to make decisions about your needs.

   2) As a manager, you first do all that you can for yourself. Second, you instruct and manage others in providing physical assistance primarily for those needs which you truly cannot perform for yourself.

The most common setting for using PCA help is in one's private housing. That setting may be in the form of a house, apartment, condominium, or cooperative apartment.

Whether the setting provides a short or long term living arrangement, the main advantages include the privacy felt within one's own "castle," the comfort of surroundings which are familiar as well as those which can be ideally modified to any architectural access needs, and the choice of live-in company to include relatives, spouse, or friends. In short, one's private home has the greatest potential for comfortable living due to a customized living environment.

If you need physical assistance, the typical contacts within your home can include relatives, spouse, lover, aide (from either an agency or personal recruiting), or a friend. At the same time, you have the on-request support of physicians, visiting nurses, and other health professionals by phone or appointment.

The titles of your relationship with those who provide assistance are a mixture of patient and manager. The title and role of patient applies to brief times when you need medical care for nonroutine ailments, as well as for physical assistance to routine needs when you are either unable or unwilling to manage for yourself. For the majority of time, you should be managing the physical assistance you require.

Many people are able to manage their own care, but well-meaning relatives and friends often interfere with this. It is common for relatives and friends at home to insist on performing many duties for you that you can do for yourself, or they may in fact wish to provide all of your physical assistance. In these situations, you may therefore feel pressure which prevents you from hiring outside PCA help.

Assistance from relatives may be very comfortable to initially accept, but in due time it will not be available to you for any of several reasons. After some time, relatives become tired of providing help day-after-day-after-day, or at least in being your only source of help...regardless of the sweet things they tell you to the contrary. In addition, the situation will not last forever because young relatives grow up and move away to conduct their own private lives; older relatives become older and can no longer meet the physical demands of assisting you. Other relatives, a spouse, or a friend also need free time to pursue their own interests, educational or career desires, or simply to have private time to themselves.

Two cautions should therefore be stated here:

> 1) <u>Do</u> insist that you be allowed to do all that you can for yourself, and that you be able to hire outside PCA assistance for at least some of your other needs, and therefore

2) <u>Do not</u> give into pressure from those around you who insist on performing tasks for you which you can do for yourself, or who insist on supplying all of the physical assistance which you require for other needs.

Your insistence in doing all that you can for yourself and hiring outside help for at least a portion of other needs may be met with resistance or even resentment by parents, relatives, a spouse, and others around you. The common reasons for this are centered around someone's assumption that you are sick and therefore unable to manage your needs, or that your seeming rejection of their help is a rejection of their love for you.

Your desire to manage your own needs might also be met with resistance by visiting aides or nurses. These people often do not encounter individuals who are knowledgeable about and want to manage their own care. They may believe you are sick and therefore incapable of making your own decisions.

These situations should be discussed in an open manner. Explain your reasons for wanting to do things for yourself and hiring outside help for other needs. Talk to those who are misunderstanding your capabilities & assertively state the reasons behind your desire to manage while showing them your knowledgeable ability to do so. Explain that the physical impairment to part of your body does not affect your overall health or your ability to think clearly and therefore it does not affect your ability to manage your own needs.

Assure your relatives that you want their continued love and that there will still be many opportunities for them to do things for you, however you wish to be self-sufficient -- just as they wish to be, themselves -- in doing certain things for yourself.

Setting: College Residence Hall or Voc-Tech/Campus Area Housing

Purpose
Short or long term living while pursuing educational/vocational training toward a job or career

Typical Contacts for Care and Assistance
Aide (from a home health agency or personal recruiting), spouse, friend, fellow student

Titles of Your Relationship to Those Who Provide Assistance
Manager, for assistance required for your routine personal needs

Your Role in This Relationship
As a manager, you first do all that you can for yourself. Second, you instruct and manage others in providing physical assistance primarily for those needs which you truly cannot perform for yourself.

There are several types of educational facilities that provide the additional education required for today's very competitive employment market. These educational facilities include vocational-technical schools, community/junior colleges, and universities. Today's student often has a choice of attending a non-residential or residential institution.

Some institutions do not provide their own housing for students. Students either live within commuting distance to their classes or they find nearby housing on their own.

Many individuals who have a recent disability, and who are still learning to manage the disability and the required PCA help, welcome the opportunity to commute from home to a nearby community or junior college program. This is especially true during their first year of adjustment to academic responsibilities. After this successful year of bite-sized responsibilities they have sharpened their PCA management skills; they have proven their academic abilities to themselves, to their relatives, and to the state's office for vocational rehabilitation (their educational funding source); and they are ready to tackle a residential program at a different campus. Some students wait to complete their 2-year associate degree before moving away from home for further studies at a 4-year institution. Others pursue a job or career for which the 2-year associate degree has adequately prepared them.

For those who decide to live away from home, there are 2 main options: to live in private housing near the voc-tech school or college campus, or to choose an institution which provides housing at its school or campus. Private housing has been discussed in the previous section of this text.

The campus might refer to its housing as either "residence halls," the more proper term, or "dormitories," from the French verb "dormer" -- hence, a place to sleep. Regardless, the objective for living in a "dorm" is to pursue educational or vocational training toward a job or career; it may be difficult to believe, but the often talked-about pizza parties are meant to be a second priority!

The primary contacts for PCA help at a campus are an aide (usually from personal recruiting) or a spouse, if the campus offers married student housing. The prime sources for personally recruiting aides are the friends and fellow students around you, although a few students use professional aides supplied by community agencies for at least some of their needs. The college campus is one of the all-time best recruiting markets, since college students are young and physically fit, flexible in their personal schedules, and looking for ways to earn money. Often a college campus will feature a department or office with a title such as "disabled student services," "disability services," or "handicapped student center." You should feel free to ask these professional staffers for advice or help in recruiting PCAs from students or surrounding community. We will discuss the college student market in more detail in chapter 24, "Sources for Recruiting PCAs."

Clearly, your title and role toward this help is as a manager. We have discussed the manager title and role in previous settings. The college campus is no place for someone who passively wishes to be a dependent patient and have others make decisions for him.

Settings in Which You Use Help

You are the direct manager of the PCA assistance which you require, unless you need a PCA Coordinator because of the inability to readily verbally communicate or meet some of the physical or visual requirements of direct management. For more details on using a PCA Coordinator, see chapter 4, "The 3 Management Situations."

Setting: Day or Evening Travel

Purpose
Short duration travel for medical and other types of appointments or meetings, educational or career responsibilities, or cultural-recreational-leisure-social activities

Typical Contacts for Care and Assistance
Aide (usually from personal recruiting), spouse, relative, friend, passer-by, or staff member of a store, library, or commercial transportation carrier

Titles of Your Relationship to Those Who Provide Assistance
Manager, for assistance required for your routine personal needs

Your Role in This Relationship
As a manager, you first do all that you can for yourself. Second, you instruct and manage others in providing physical assistance primarily for those needs which you truly cannot perform for yourself.

As mentioned before, few of us wish to live our entire lives within the four walls of our living area. There are medical appointments, many types of meetings, meals at restaurants, education and career responsibilities, church services, shopping and banking needs, romantic dates, and a huge variety of cultural, recreational, leisure, and social activities which we may want to enjoy.

The objective of day and evening travel is short duration travel which does not require an overnight stay away from one's own home. Day and evening travel can be of any distance, whether a walk around the block to get a quart of milk or a day-long business meeting at a conference 400 miles away which requires a round trip flight in the same day on a commuters air shuttle.

The typical contacts for any assistance required includes an aide (usually from personal recruiting), spouse, relative, friend, brief help from a passer-by, or the staff of a store, library, or commercial transportation carrier. Assistance can come from a PCA who is with us the entire time, or from a stranger whom we briefly encounter. After all, many of us would find everyday independence considerably more difficult or limited if friendly passers-by or the staff in stores or airlines weren't available to offer help with such quick, nonpersonal needs as

- cumbersome store entrance doors
- grocery items, cafeteria food, or library books which are out-of-reach on high or low shelves
- grocery sacks which are too heavy, numerous, or fragile for carrying by wheelchair to one's car
- cafeteria/fast food trays with hot and spillable coffee or tea
- heavy baggage to be carried through the "miles" of airport gates
- other cars which park too close to one's own to enable wheelchair transfer or using one's van lift.

Your title and role toward this assistance is clearly that of a manager, as we have discussed in previous settings. A few exceptions to the manager role might occur for very dependent individuals who travel on a specially planned private trip or group tour with a close friend, relative, spouse, or medical personnel.

You are the direct manager of the PCA assistance which you require, unless you need a PCA Coordinator because of the inability to readily verbally communicate or meet some of the physical or visual requirements of directly managing. For more details on using a PCA Coordinator, see chapter 4, "The 3 Management Situations."

Setting: Overnight Travel

Purpose
Short/long term or distance travel for any reason via car, camper, bus, air, rail, or ship

Typical Contacts for Care and Assistance
Aide (usually from personal recruiting), spouse, relative, friend, passer-by, or staff member of a store, lodging establishment, or commercial transportation carrier

Titles of Your Relationship to Those Who Provide Assistance
Manager, for assistance required for your routine personal needs

Your Role in This Relationship
As a manager, you first do all that you can for yourself. Second, you instruct and manage others in providing physical assistance primarily for those needs which you truly cannot perform for yourself.

When day-travel vacations do not provide sufficient relaxation, or when educational or career responsibilities require a 3-day conference in a far city, then overnight travel might be necessary.

The purpose for overnight travel is for either short or long term travel, of either a short or long distance, for any reason. Transportation might be provided by car, camper, van, bus, air, rail, or ship. Lodging can be at a $ 300 per day luxury resort: small roadside motel; ski resort (in or out of season); campsite within an ocean, mountain, forest, desert, or fishing stream setting; private and accessible Amtrak sleeper car; guest room on a cruise ship; RV or pop-up camper, or at a neighborhood friend's house.

The available help usually comes from an aide (usually from personal recruiting), spouse, relative, friend, or brief help from a passer-by or the staff help from a store, lodging accommodation, or commercial carrier.

Your title and role toward this help in this independent setting is usually, once more, as a manager. A few exceptions to the manager role might occur for very dependent patients who travel on a specially planned private trip or group tour with a close friend, relative, spouse, or medical personnel.

You are the direct manager of the PCA assistance which you require, unless you need a PCA Coordinator because of the inability to readily verbally communicate or meet some of the physical or visual requirements of direct management. For more details on using a PCA Coordinator, see chapter 4, "The 3 Management Situations."

7. Types of Help & the Services Each Provider Performs

Listed in the following 3-section chart are three primary types of help from which many of us frequently receive services. Each type differs in the kinds of services it will provide and the cost of the assistance. It is important that you know where to find each type of help, the kinds of services available from each type of help, strategies for taking maximum advantage of each service, and the comparative costs to you or your funding source.

I
Type of Help: Health Professionals Working at Institutions

Typical Titles: Physician, Nurse, Nursing Assistant, Aide, Therapist, Counselor, Social Worker

Previous Professional Training?: Yes, extensive

Services You Can Receive: Diagnosis, Development of treatment plan, Medical care & therapies, Education and Counseling about your ailment or disability & your responsibilities toward care & rehabilitation, Follow-up visits & advice by phone

---

II
Type of Help: Health Professionals Working in Your Home Who are Provided by Agencies

Agency Categories: Commercial, Government Sponsored, Non-Profit

Typical Titles: Registered Nurse (RN), Licensed Practical Nurse (LPN), Nursing Assistant, Home Health Aide, Personal Care Aide/Attendant (PCA), Homemaker, Companion, Others

Previous Professional Training?: Yes, ranges from several years of formal training to briefings on interpersonal skills. Regardless of any prior training, all providers will require instructions about your specific needs and probably some degree of on-site management, quality control, and supervision from you or your designate.

Services You Can Receive:
1) Medical care for nonroutine ailments, and
2) Physical assistance for routine needs

III

Type of Help: Health Professionals & Others Working in Your Home Whom You Personally Recruit & Directly Employ

Typical Titles: RN, LPN, Nursing Assistant, Home Health Aide, Personal Care Aide/Attendant (PCA), Housekeeper, Homemaker, Companion, Sitter, Transportation Driver, Maintenance Worker, Volunteer

Previous Professional Training?: Yes & No, some may have received extensive training while others will be trained completely by you. Regardless of any prior training, all providers will require instructions about your specific needs and on-site management, quality control, and supervision from you or your designate.

Services You Can Receive:
1) Medical care for nonroutine ailments, and
2) Physical assistance for routine needs

94   Types of Help & the Services Each Provider Performs

I
Type of Help: Health Professionals Working at Institutions

Typical Titles: Physician, Nurse, Nursing Assistant, Aide, Therapist, Counselor, Social Worker

Previous Professional Training?: Yes, extensive

Services You Can Receive: Diagnosis, Development of treatment plan, Medical care & therapies, Education and Counseling about your ailment or disability & your responsibilities toward care & rehabilitation, Follow-up visits & advice by phone

Health Professionals Working at Institutions

The first type of help listed in the chart is that available from institutional health professionals...the professionals who work in an acute care hospital, rehabilitation hospital, health care center, health maintenance organization (HMO), or clinic. To simplify our chart, we refer to seven titles of professionals with whom a patient has the most frequent contact: physician, nurse, nursing assistant, aide, therapist, counselor, and social worker. These are the professionals who provide you with the initial assessment and details, or diagnosis, of your medical concern or disability. They will also serve as an ongoing resource of medical information, and therefore provide you with the information you require to instruct PCAs about your needs. Each of these professionals has received extensive training.

Although these professionals provide a multitude of services, we have simplified our chart by listing the five primary services of special concern to our discussion, and explain how to take maximum advantage of each.

Diagnosis refers to identifying an ailment by examining and analyzing its symptoms. This process begins when you make an appointment with a health professional and say, "I have come to see you because I don't feel well." The professional then asks you for symptoms that give you the impression that something is wrong. The professional tries to fit these symptoms together in various ways like a picture puzzle until a specific picture, or in medical terms an "ailment," is identified. This can be a simple process, for a patient with a common cold, or a complex process which involves a variety of laboratory tests and scans.

Developing a treatment plan refers to the health professional deciding on a game plan for correcting the identified ailment or for minimizing the effects of a disability. This treatment can be simple, in prescribing aspirin, bedrest, and plenty of fluids for the patient with the common cold, or complex in the lengthy care and therapies of a hospital in-patient. If the decision between prescribing in- or out-patient care is a close toss-up, the physician might consider factors such as whether you can obtain a sufficient degree of medical care at home as well as your ability to manage and monitor the quality of that care while at home.

The objective of the medical care and therapies is to carry out the treatment plan in order to cure or minimize the negative effects of the ailment or disability. This process may involve your supervision of your own care at home, as a hospital out-patient, or your participation with a number of health professionals as an in-patient at an acute care hospital or rehabilitation hospital.

> You should ask sincere questions of health professionals in order to be a layman-authority on your own medical history & how your body works

The fourth primary service which you should know how to obtain from institutional health professionals is the education and counseling which these people can offer you. The objective of taking advantage of this education and guidance is to enable you to learn as much as you wish about your body and its normal functions as well as nonroutine problems. This knowledge enables you to participate with health professionals in decisions about diagnoses, treatment plans, and methods of actual medical care and therapies regarding existing problems, as well as preventative health care to minimize the recurrence of problems in the future. This knowledge is also essential for your being a good PCA manager. It gives you a basis for the methods and rationale for your own physical assistance so that you can convey that information to others who help you.

There are two steps to becoming educated about your own body and its problems. First, develop a genuine, ongoing interest in learning more about your health. Second, ask sincere questions of health professionals whenever you genuinely wish information or do not understand something about your body or methods for its care. Professionals usually welcome questions which are asked for sincere and appropriate reasons; they usually resent questions that are asked by patients who aren't sincerely interested in answers and who merely want to impress them with some kind of arrogant authority. If your questions come from a genuine interest to learn ways of living a more healthy life, then the health professional usually will be glad to provide clear answers.

When should you feel free to ask questions? Situations include the following:

▌ During the diagnosis, regarding the basic facts and symptoms which identify your ailment or disability,

▌ During the development of the treatment plan, for understanding why your physician is prescribing a specific plan of medical care as well as understanding the details and procedures for that care and therapy,

▌ During the actual performance of medical care and therapies, to monitor the quality of care and to compare the type and schedule of treatment that you receive with the original treatment plan which was prescribed,

▌ For in-patients, to determine what post-discharge responsibilities you have for providing or managing your own medical care after you leave the hospital,

▌ For out-patients, to determine what home-based responsibilities you have for providing or managing your own medical care,

▌ After symptoms of the ailment have disappeared or minimized, to determine what follow-up responsibilities you have for arranging further medical checkups, and

Types of Help & the Services Each Provider Performs 97

■ At anytime by phone or office appointment, to ask questions for advice whenever you have concerns about caring for a new ailment or about old methods of performing care for a routine need.

II

Type of Help: Health Professionals Working in Your Home Who are Provided by Agencies

Agency Categories: Commercial, Government Sponsored, Non-Profit

Typical Titles: Registered Nurse (RN), Licensed Practical Nurse (LPN), Nursing Assistant, Home Health Aide, Personal Care Aide/Attendant (PCA), Homemaker, Companion, Others

Previous Professional Training?: Yes, ranges from several years of formal training to briefings on interpersonal skills. Regardless of any prior training, all providers will require instructions about your specific needs and probably some degree of on-site management, quality control, and supervision from you or your designate.

Services You Can Receive:
1) Medical care for nonroutine ailments, and
2) Physical assistance for routine needs

Health Professionals Working in Your Home Who are Provided by Agencies

The type of help listed in chart II is that provided by professionals who are both employed and insured against malpractice by an agency. There are several categories of agencies such as the commercial agencies found in most telephone yellow pages, the government sponsored agencies such as public, state, county, or city health departments, and a few nonprofit agencies which may charge minimal fees on a sliding scale to cover basic expenses.

> Compare the primary factors of using either agency-provided or personally-employed help, and use the type which better matches your abilities & desires

In any case, an agency's role is to recruit, interview, schedule, pay, otherwise manage, and sometimes train professionals on behalf of the actual recipient of services.

Types of Help & the Services Each Provider Performs   99

Agencies perform an essential set of services for certain individuals who a) are unwilling or unable to manage their own care, or b) receive funding for services and are required by their funding source to seek assistance from certain approved agencies. Some recipients also validly use an agency's services for a temporary period of time until they are later able or willing to manage assistance for themselves.

Some primary advantages and disadvantages of using agency services are further discussed in the "Comparisons" section which appears after the next discussion of Chart III.

Types of Help & the Services Each Provider Performs

III
<u>Type of Help</u>: Health Professionals & Others Working in Your Home Whom You Personally Recruit & Directly Employ

<u>Typical Titles</u>: RN, LPN, Nursing Assistant, Home Health Aide, Personal Care Aide/Attendant (PCA), Housekeeper, Homemaker, Companion, Sitter, Transportation Driver, Maintenance Worker, Volunteer

<u>Previous Professional Training?</u>: Yes & No, some may have received extensive training while others will be trained completely by you. Regardless of any prior training, all providers will require instructions about your specific needs and on-site management, quality control, and supervision from you or your designate.

<u>Services You Can Receive:</u>
1) Medical care for nonroutine ailments, and
2) Physical assistance for routine needs

Health Professionals & Others Working in Your Home Whom You Personally Recruit & Directly Employ

The type of help listed in chart III includes those people whom you, by yourself, recruit, interview and screen, schedule, train, and pay regarding your own needs. Obtaining help in this way requires that you be able and willing to directly manage and otherwise employ the assistance which you need. These abilities can be learned from the topic-by-topic information in this book. Beyond the textbook details of this book, PCA management abilities are fine tuned, as within any field of management, through years of trial, error, and practice. Most folks have found that the numerous advantages of being a self-sufficient manager are well worth the efforts of learning and practice.

Listed below are some of the primary considerations for deciding whether to use agency-provided help or personally-employed help.

Comparisons: Should You Use Agency-Provided Help or Personally-Recruited Help in Your Home?

In deciding whether to use services which are coordinated and employed by an agency, or those which you directly employ, you should consider at least seven factors: your willingness to be a manager, costs, training, the range of duties that must be performed, the choice of personnel, providing different types of employment insurance, and observing requirements of employment records and taxes. Each of these are examined in detail.

Your Willingness and Ability to Be a Manager   A major determining factor between using help which is coordinated and employed by an agency or directly employed by you is your degree of willingness and ability to assume, yourself, the managerial responsibilities.

As mentioned previously, many folks are unwilling or unable to manage assistance. Those unable to do so include recipients of services who lack the emotional stability or intellectual ability required for assessing their own needs and then proceding to recruit, train, and manage providers who can supply them required assistance.

Others are able but unwilling to be managers and have, for some reason, chosen not to want to be in managerial control of the help which they use. For those with a short-term, homebound recovery from an ailment, sometimes there is an understandable lack of desire to learn and practice management skills for such a seemingly temporary need for assistance. For others with a longer-term or supposedly life-long disability, sometimes the rejection of becoming a self-sufficient manager is consistent with their rejection of accepting their disability. Consequently, they refuse to assume the responsibility for coordinating their own care. For either of these cases, an agency's coordination and management of professional help is essential.

For those who are unable or unwilling to manage, an agency's coordination and management of professional assistance is essential. If, however, the recipient of services or his personal designate is able and willing to directly manage assistance, a list of advantageous controls over that assistance will be realized. These advantages are discussed in the next topics of this section.

Costs An agency charges you, or your funding source, both for the hourly salary which it pays the actual PCA as well as for the administrative fee which it charges for its management tasks. For example, if you use assistance from a home health aide, the agency might pay that aide an hourly salary of $ 5.50. However, the total hourly rate which is billed to you includes an additional administrative fee which can range from a few dollars to over $ 20.00 per hour.

Cost of Using Agency = Hourly Salary Which the Agency Pays the Provider +Administrative Overhead & Fees
Cost of Directly Employing Help = Hourly Salary Which You Pay the Provider + Possible Taxes

If you receive third party funding for medical help at home, the funding source might require you to use an agency which has their approval. This stipulation often exists, in part, so that the funding source is assured that you receive services from trained and certified personnel.

If you are unwilling or unable, on a temporary or permanent basis, to manage and employ assistance on your own, or if your funding source requires you to use agency-employed help, then you will find that using agency services is essential. However, if you are paying for assistance from your own pocket and you are willing and able to manage assistance yourself, then the savings you will realize over a period of time on directly employing help and avoiding agency administrative fees can be enormous...as much as $ 20.00 per hour!

Training If you use an agency's help, you are assured that the personnel have been trained and usually certified to the extent required by the title which each individual staff member holds. The agency may or may not have provided this training itself.

Types of Help & the Services Each Provider Performs 103

All nurses must have extensive training and be certified by the state in which they practice, whether they work for an institution, an agency, or for an individual. A nurse usually graduates from a school or college before they can register with one or several agencies. A nursing assistant or aide employed by an agency must also graduate from a formal training program and receive a certification, although such training is considerably less than that of a nurse. In some agencies, there are several types of aides and homemakers and each receives a different level of training; consequently, each type of personnel is allowed by the agency to perform very specific duties which are appropriate to their particular level of training. Some agencies will provide this training for aides or subcontract the task to a training school, while other agencies do not train but require that new aide employees provide a document of proof that they have completed training and certification.

If you decide to directly employ your own assistance, you can still tap into help providers who have completed the same training and certification required by agencies. The recruiting you conduct (which can include placing ads in newspapers and other methods explained in chapter 25, "Methods for Recruiting PCAs") can attract responses from trained nurses and aides. These folks may be working part or full time for an institution or agency and may be willing to also work for you in their spare hours. Thus, you will be using the same fully trained providers who would be supplied by an agency, but you will be paying an hourly salary only to the provider without the additional administrative fee charged by agencies for their management expenses.

In addition to using trained providers, you might choose to employ help providers who have not received any previous training. Many of us have successfully employed untrained and inexperienced assistance for many years from the students of a nearby college campus as well as other types of help which are listed in chapter 24, "Sources for Recruiting PCAs."

This untrained help can be successfully used only if the assistance is not of a complex medical nature that requires trained nursing help. In addition, you, the recipient of services -- and direct employer of help -- must have skills of an effective trainer in addition to being an effective manager. This book offers you both kinds of skills; all that is additionally needed is practice. Many people who routinely require physical assistance have never used previously trained aides, and have simply instructed recruited help with regard to fulfilling their particular needs.

> Whether the help you use is formally trained or inexperienced, they will ask for instruction about your particular needs

After all, one must provide much of the same instruction for meeting one's particular needs to either trained or untrained help, regardless of whether that help comes through an agency or personal recruiting. Using agency-trained help might slightly lessen the need for management skills on your part, but certainly does not totally relieve you of the need to know and use these skills. Both agency-provided and personally-recruited help will make the same statement on the first day you use them, "OK, here I am; please tell me what kinds of assistance you need, and how and on what schedule you want me to provide that assistance."

<u>Range of Duties</u> Each type of service provider from an agency has completed a level of formal training appropriate to their title. For example, a registered nurse has more training than a home health aide. Consequently, a registered nurse is allowed by the agency to perform more medically complex duties than an aide is permitted to perform. Some agencies have separate titles for a home health aide, personal care aide, and homemaker. Again, each title of provider receives a different level of training and is allowed to perform only types of work appropriate to the training received.

If you have a wide range of needs for which physical assistance is required, you may be frustrated to discover that agency-provided help is not allowed by the agency to perform certain duties. This wide range of duties might include assistance with medical needs, housecleaning, doing laundry, help in stores with shopping, driving one's personal transportation, and simple household

Types of Help & the Services Each Provider Performs

maintenance. In some cases, 2 or 3 types of help must be hired through an agency to cover the entire range of duties; in other cases where funding or other restrictions prevent hiring 2 or 3 types of help, certain needs for assistance must go unfulfilled.

This strict hierarchy of duties is due, in part, to the agency's responsibility to its malpractice insurance carrier. The agency must guarantee the insurance carrier that each provider is sufficiently trained for duties being performed. In addition, some agencies and the funding sources which pay those agencies on your behalf do not want to pay an aide for duties which they consider to be beyond your basic medical needs...regardless of how important those tasks are to you.

Below are 3 job descriptions which illustrate the duties which one agency actually permits three titles of its providers to perform. Job descriptions vary among agencies and those cited below should be considered merely as illustrations which compare the permitted functions of the 3 positions.

Registered Nurse (RN)

An RN tends to the physical and psycho-social needs of the patient and his/her family.

Functions
1. Assist with the development and implementation of the nursing care plan which is received from the physician.
2. Assist all other medically-related, personal care activities.
3. Administer medication prescribed by the physician.
4. Instruct patient and family in self-care procedures as indicated.
5. Perform all treatments as prescribed by the physician.
6. Maintain safe environment.
7. Perform nursing procedures as experience has demonstrated and as permitted by the Nurse Practice Act.
8. Maintain documentation on all nursing activities and assessments.

Home Care
1. Report patient changes to RN Supervisor.
2. Submit weekly "nurse's notes" to the agency office.
3. Perform household tasks directly related to patient's health:

   a) Maintain clean environment
   b) Meal preparation
   c) Maintain patient care equipment

Qualifications
1. Current state RN license
2. Minimum one year's experience working as an RN

Licensed Practical Nurse (LPN)

The LPN works under the guidance and supervision of a Registered Nurse and performs nursing procedures where a professional degree of evaluative judgement is not required.

Functions
1. Assists with the preparation, implementation, and continuing evaluation of the nursing plan.
2. Assists patient with cleanliness, grooming, rest, nourishment, and elimination.

Types of Help & the Services Each Provider Performs

3. Maintains a safe environment.
4. Performs specific treatments as ordered by the physician.
5. Administers medications and treatments prescribed by the physician.
6. Observes, records, and reports to the appropriate nursing supervisor or physician any symptoms, reactions, and changes including:

   a) general physical and mental condition of patients as well as signs and symptoms which may be indicative of changes
   b) stresses in patient and/or family relationships

Home Care
1. Report changes to the RN Supervisor.
2. Submit weekly "nurse's notes" to the agency.
3. Perform incidental household tasks essential to the patient's well being:

   a) Maintain patient care equipment
   b) Maintain clean environment
   c) Meal preparation

Patient Care Activities Not Permitted by Agency
1. Initial patient assessments.
2. Administration of experimental medications or desensitization drugs

Qualifications
1. Current state LPN license
2. Minimum of one year's experience working as an LPN

Nursing Assistant/Home Health Aide

The following is a guideline of the duties which you are permitted to perform in the home. You will have a nursing plan in the home which outlines your patient's needs, as determined by the physician and your RN Supervisor. You will work under the direction of your RN Supervisor.

Functions
1. Assist with bathing the patient - sponge, bed, shower, tub.
2. Assist with grooming - shampoo and comb hair, shaving, nail care (filing and cleaning, only).
3. Assist with care of teeth, dentures, mouth.

4. Assist with dressing.
5. Assist with eating, prepare and serve normal diets.
6. Assist with toileting - on and off commode, toilet, or bedpan; provide and remove urinal.
7. Assist with positioning in bed - moving from bed to chair, to wheelchair, and in walking.
8. Remind patient to follow medical recommendations as written on nursing care plan.
9. Complete aide worksheet daily as instructed on the care plan.
10. Perform incidental, light household tasks to maintain a safe and healthy environment for the patient:

Functions You May Not Perform
1. Cutting nails - fingers or toes
2. Administer enema
3. Change sterile dressings
4. Colostomy irrigation
5. Apply heat
6. Administer medications
7. Gastric gavage
8. Tracheostomy tube care
9. Vaginal douche
10. Indwelling catheter irrigation
11. Make medical or nursing judgements, give medical advice, or call physician
12. Give injections
13. Give rectal or vaginal suppositories
14. Heavy household tasks: mopping floors, washing windows, cleaning refrigerators or stove/oven areas, dusting or vacuuming which is not within the patient's room, laundry which is either not the patient's or which must be done outside the immediate premises, or outdoor maintenance and cleaning activities

If you directly employ the assistance you use, there are few restrictions on the types of duties which a provider can perform for you. The primary limitations are these:

a) Your choice of duties for a provider should match the mental and physical abilities of the provider as well as your ability to adequately instruct the provider. For example, few of us would trust the ability of an aide, or our own ability to instruct an aide, in the correct or safe procedures for draining or dressing an infected pressure sore for the first time -- such requires the medical skills of a physician or nurse.,

b) The agreement from the aide to perform a particular duty. In answer to your asking a directly employed aide, "Would you be willing to do such-and-such?," an aide always has the right to say, "No, I would rather not.", and

c) Your choice of matching an appropriate category of provider with an appropriate category of duty. For example, it would be a waste of the highly trained skills and high hourly salary of a registered nurse to ask her to wash, dry, and fold laundry or to mop floors and wash windows, however such would be appropriate duties for an aide, homemaker, or housekeeper whom you employ.

With these limitations in mind, the PCA you directly employ can be requested -- not ordered -- to do almost anything. In return, their right to refuse must be respected.

<u>Choice of Personnel, Schedule, Quality, & Sick Time Replacements</u> An agency recruits, interviews, screens, schedules, supervises, fires, and sometimes trains providers on behalf of the actual recipients of services. "On behalf of" means that the agency -- and not you -- creates guideline policies and makes decisions which determine who assists you, their qualifications, their schedule for arriving and departing from your home, and whether poor performance will be repeatedly tolerated or promptly considered grounds for replacing the aide.

> Agency-provided help is essential to many people, however it brings unnecessary costs and restrictions to those who can personally employ help

If you are unable or unwilling to manage and directly employ assistance, these agency functions are essential. These service recipients inform the agency of the frequency and time schedule for which assistance is needed. The agency checks its listings of nurses and aides who are available to work that frequency and schedule, and otherwise does its best to assure that a nurse or aide will arrive on schedule at the recipient's home. Sometimes the

110   Types of Help & the Services Each Provider Performs

availability of aides does not match the desired schedule of the service recipient, and the recipient is notified by the agency regarding the adjusted schedule which the aides will actually maintain.

You should also realize that an agency manytimes schedules a service provider to visit several recipients each day, one after the other. This cost efficient system works well until one of the recipients on a provider's list has an unexpected need which takes extra time, for example a bowel accident. Agency supplied service providers have been known to handle the situation in either of two ways: to leave the recipient on schedule with some details unfinished, or to finish all scheduled details and be late for each of their next appointments. In the former case, each recipient receives assistance on schedule, but one recipient is left for the day without all of her scheduled needs fulfilled. In the second case, the provider takes the extra time required to complete expected duties but is consequently late for each subsequent appointment that day. Anyone who is considering the use of an agency should inquire about the agency's policy regarding such a situation.

On the occasion that a scheduled service provider is sick or otherwise unable to provide expected assistance, some agencies have readily available replacements...others do not. In many geographical areas, the supply of available aides is not sufficient or an agency simply does not maintain an adequate list of backup aides. Consequently, some agencies have trouble filling even initial client requests with "first string" help. When a routinely scheduled, first stringer is suddenly sick, some agencies are unable to provide replacements. The agency returns to its own listing -- or a "free-lance" listing -- of aides and places phone calls with the hope of finding a fill-in. This task becomes additionally difficult because aides are often not employed on a full time basis by any single agency and therefore the aides usually free-lance and register for work with more than one agency. Consequently, few agencies can count on an aide being available for unexpected work when needed. If you are considering the use of a particular agency, ask in advance about how promptly sick time replacements are routinely made, and if there have been circumstances when no replacement has been possible.

Types of Help & the Services Each Provider Performs   111

We mentioned that many agencies are operating within a geographical area where there is a shortage of available aides. If an agency has difficulty in initially filling your schedule, and has additional difficulty in promptly finding sick time replacements, then it will also have difficulty in replacing an aide with whom you are not satisfied This dissatisfaction can come from a poor quality of work, a frequently poor schedule of arrival and departure times, an inability or lack of desire of an aide to follow reasonable instructions from you, or indeed unethical behavior. In such circumstances, you are not the direct employer and you lack the authority that the agency possesses since it, alone, is the source of the aide's paycheck. You can complain to the aide about problems, however if complaints are ignored by the aide, you must plead your case to the agency. Some agencies are prompt to remedy a problem situation and replace an aide if necessary, and some agencies are not.

If you are the direct manager and employer of assistance which you use, you have much more authority and control over each of these situations. You are in a position to hire and fire directly employed assistance, and the PCA quickly recognizes this authority. Your control applies to the discussed situations of:

a) Controlling the schedule of assistance which you receive because you hire only those PCAs who agree to meet the exact schedule which is required by your activities,

b) Controlling the schedule of assistance which you receive because the PCA is not shared with other service recipients,

c) Controlling the prompt sick time replacement of PCAs because you maintain an adequate list of backups, and you might employ several part-time PCAs instead of entrusting all of your needs with just one PCA, and

d) Controlling or remedying the bad habits, or firing and replacing uncooperative PCAs, because as a direct employer you have the authority to do so as needed.

Of course, controlling all of these factors is a considerable responsibility and necessitates careful management. There are no guarantees that a good manager will be successful in controlling all of these factors, but the direct manager will have at least the opportunity to attempt to do so. Most private PCA managers will agree that having the opportunity for those controls over the quality and schedule of the help they receive is well worth the effort.

> Personally employing help requires considerable planning & responsibility, but also gives you maximum control over the quality of assistance which you receive

Insurance There are 3 types of insurance which agencies provide: 1) malpractice insurance, 2) workers' compensation and disability benefits insurances, and 3) unemployment insurance.

Malpractice insurance is provided by most agencies for their employees so that, in the event that an employed aide causes harm to a recipient because of negligence or unprofessional performance, the service recipient may collect a monetary compensation for the harm done from the insurance instead of from the assets of either the agency or the aide.

Malpractice insurance is carried by many highly trained medical professionals, such as physicians, therapists, and nurses. These individuals are either required to have such insurance by their employer or they usually choose to be covered at their own expense in order to protect their personal assets from a potential law suit. Many aides and homemakers, however, cannot personally afford such insurance and therefore are not covered unless the insurance is supplied by their employer.

Since a malpractice suit would usually involve the employer, most agencies choose to provide insurance for their employees in order to protect the agency's own assets. If an aide is directly employed by an individual, and the aide does not personally carry malpractice insurance, then the aide's personal assets could be sued by the individual who has experienced harm from the aide's negligence. However, since the value of most people's personal assets would not adequately reimburse a successful half-million dollar law suit, there would be little point in attempting to sue such an individual aide. Hence, the direct, private employer takes a risk that the performance of an aide will not be negligent and cause harm.

The private employer minimizes the chance for harm to occur by carefully instructing and supervising aides in the quality of their work. The aides are instructed in the proper and safe methods for performing duties, and quality control is exercised by the employer to be sure the safe methods are consistently followed and that the procedures do not become sloppy. In addition, direct employers are very quick to fire and replace any PCA who repeatedly performs duties in a hazardous way, or who at anytime attempts to perform duties while under the influence of drugs or alcohol.

Workers' compensation insurance pays an employee medical benefits and a portion of their salary for the duration of an illness or injury which is caused by their job or which occurs on their job site. Disability benefits insurance pays a portion of salary to an employee during an illness or injury which is not job-related.

Both of these closely related insurances are often required by state laws, and the employer purchases the insurance by paying periodic premiums to a commercial carrier of their choice. The requirements, which are stipulated by state law, vary from state to state and can be obtained by calling any state's department of labor.

In some states, a home health aide agency is required to supply the insurances for employees, however the private individual who will be personally employing aides in his home as domestic help often is not required to provide these particular insurances when "domestic ('around the house') employees are employed less than 40 hours per week." Check your own state's requirements.

Many renters or homeowners will find that limited workers' compensation coverage is included in their renter's or homeowner's insurance coverage. An increasing number of policies are including workman's compensation insurance for part time employees who are employed at a residence for non-commercial, not-for-profit purposes. So if your policy includes this coverage, and a PCA injures himself while physically helping you or mowing your lawn, you might be covered for the medical expenses incurred by your employee. Check your policy.

With regard to unemployment insurance, there are both federal and state requirements. Agencies are required to pay this insurance, while often individuals who personally employ their own aides for a small number of hours are not required to do so. Details about unemployment insurance are provided in chapter 19, "Tax Obligations for A PCA Employer."

Employment Records and Taxes If you use agency-provided help, these requirements, and associated employer tax expenses, are the responsibility of the agency. If you are the employer, the responsibilities are yours. These and other employer responsibilities are included in chapter 19, "Tax Obligations for A PCA Employer."

8. Qualities and Strategies of a Good Manager

In this section, you will find simplified, but very important versions of some primary strategies used by all good managers...not used by all managers, but all good ones. "Good help is hard to find," and if you ignore these strategies, you will fail time after time to keep good help for very long. If you ignore these strategies, good help will not want to stay with you...we guarrantee it!

First, some definitions.

There have been many books written, and many university courses and seminars taught, on various theories of management. These theories have been studied by small business owners as well as top corporate executives. Executives often manage hundreds of employees in multi-million dollar industries; retired folks often quietly manage household help. Everyone who employs and manages assistance should learn at least the basic strategies of being the type of manager for whom people want to work.

Whether the management situation involves thousands of employees or a single gardener doing household chores, the main objective for which every manager aims is "to have employees perform assigned duties in the most efficient way possible." In turn, "efficient" can be defined as "providing the highest possible quality and quantity of work for the lowest possible cost."

If you manage the PCAs whom you use, then you want a high quality of assistance for a quantity of time which is sufficient to enable you to maintain your own personal schedule.

> The "positive management approach" results in employees who want to work hard for you and who don't feel forced to do so

The trick is to receive this type of assistance in return for the lowest possible costs to you and to the PCA who helps you. Costs to you include the time and effort which you spend performing your duties as a manager, plus the amount of salary which you pay the PCA. Costs to the PCA include mostly the time and effort which are spent in giving you assistance.

There are several classically bad and good strategies used by managers. Most of the bad strategies are selfishly chosen and stubbornly kept by bad managers because they become blind to the negative effects of their bad habits on employees. Their egos tell them that "good and powerful managers" have always used such strategies. Even if they do recognize their faults, they do not often know how to correct them or how to adopt better management methods.

You can be different.

A traditional, outdated image that some employers have is that a supervisor or boss must command respect from employees by constantly appearing to be authoritative and powerful. "Don't let the workers get an upper hand," and "Give them and inch and they'll take a yard" are two old sayings which seem to prove that employees "can't be trusted" and must be "kept in line."

Perhaps these concepts are carry overs from the use of slave labor, however they are not at all in keeping with the methods of a more modern managerial school which emphasizes maintaining mutual respect between employers and employees. There are two primary management styles which we are discussing here. Poor managers who do not know any better tend to be rude and rule over an employee in order to *force* the employee to work and work faster (the "forceful approach"); the smart manager provides a pleasant work environment in which employees *want* to work (the "positive approach").

The forceful approach. The erroneous and traditional way of "motivating" a donkey which is hitched to a cart is to hit or whip the animal in order to keep it moving. The manager who adopts this traditional style feels that he is powerful and in command by conditioning the animal to perform tasks in order to avoid pain, and that punishment occurs whenever the animal doesn't perform as desired. When the animal sees the trainer or hears him yell, the animal jumps from a sense of fear, resulting in the trainer falsely believing that he is a respected authority. Many donkeys would tell you that they don't really respect or like working for such a trainer who is so cruel; many human employees will tell you the same thing about working for a similar type of employer.

In using the donkey illustration as a management model, we can easily see that many employers -- whose egos are over inflated and whose skills are limited -- find that they have little contact with employees unless there comes a need to discipline or reprimand them for doing something wrong. These poor quality managers depend upon rudeness as a strategy for showing their authority. "Rudeness" has been defined by smart managers as "a weak man's way of showing power."

The forceful approach is loaded with disadvantages to both the boss and employees. It results in employees who resent the boss as much as the work which they are performing under constant stress. Like the donkey whose only reason to work is to avoid the sting of the whip, the predominant reason for these human employees to work is to avoid the sting of reprimands and verbal abuse from their boss. As soon as the trainer is absent, the donkey knows that he won't be whipped and he often slows or stops working until he hears the trainer coming back. As soon as a forceful boss is absent, the employees also tend to slow or stop work. Human employees do so both in the absence of the boss' supervision and as a way of "getting back" at a boss whom they bitterly resent. Consequently, the quality and quantity of work fluctuates with the presence and absence of the boss. Knowing this, the boss finds it necessary -- and very time consuming and tiring -- to spend most of his time being present and tightly supervising ("riding reign over") the employees.

In one final disadvantage of the forceful approach, the employees typically dislike or even hate their boss as well as the work which they are performing. As soon as more attractive jobs appear, the forceful boss will tend to lose employees frequently...and just as often the employees feel very little loyalty or other reason to respect their boss, and they give him very little notice of their upcoming departure. After all, what has the boss ever done to show respect for the employees?!

The positive approach. The second management approach, which we are terming the "positive approach," is loaded with advantages for both the manager and employees. Here, the smart manager doesn't _force_ the employees to work for her, but instead provides a pleasant working environment so that employees decide on their own that they _want_ to work for, and please, the manager.

A pleasant working environment is one where the manager first respects the employee, and in turn earns respect from the employee. Each of these two parties shows its respect for the other in numerous ways (see listings under the chapters "Rights for You & the PCA" and "The Top 10 Reasons Why PCAs Quit & Are Fired"). Another fairly comprehensive listing appears for you in the section of this book entitled "Job Expectations." In that section, you will find ways for both the manager and the PCA to contribute to a pleasant, smoothly running work environment...an environment where the PCA gets what she expects in a nice place to work, and where you get what you expect in high quality services of a reasonable quantity.

When you provide a pleasant work environment, the employee arrives to find that the work is easier...her duties are clearly defined, are of a reasonable nature, and the work area is efficiently layed out and well equipped. Moreover, she quickly discovers that you are a firm manager, but one who trusts each PCA to be capable of quality work unless the PCA negatively proves otherwise.

> Good managers do not force or command employee respect, they earn it by first respecting employees

There are numerous advantages to the positive approach, and consequently of an employee deciding that they want to work well and to please you. The time and effort which you spend in supervision is cut to a minimum. The quality and quantity of work is much higher than can ever be realized under the forceful method, because here both the employer and employee are working together. PCAs tend to want to keep their jobs longer, even in the sight of other jobs which pay slightly more, because they like the work which they are doing. When a PCA has been respected and does decide to

Qualities and Strategies of a Good Manager 119

quit, and she knows that an advance notice of her departure is desired by her employer, she is more inclined to give that advance notice in return for the respect she has received. She may even offer to briefly work beyond her quitting date if the manager is having problems finding a replacement.

In discussing the forceful and positive approaches, we have mentioned that mutual respect between the employer and employee is a key ingredient of the positive approach.

"Respect," simply defined, is "showing regard or consideration for another." Between an employer and employee, it means that if the employer outwardly cares about what's important to the employee, the employee will usually care about what's important to the employer. Both parties benefit.

Most of us have experienced two types of respect in our relationships with others. One type is a forced respect, which is undesirable in most employment relations. The other is earned respect, which is an integral part of the desired, positive approach to managing employees.

Forced respect results from an employer, manager, supervisor, or perhaps school teacher (!) trying to acquire respect by making others fear their power and authority. The sense of impending fear usually comes from the constant threat of some sort of punishment if respect is not shown. We can term this respect "forced," because few subordinates, employees, or students show this type of respect willingly, but because they are given the choice of showing respect or being punished.

Most armies use a sense of forced respect for ruling troops during combat conditions. It is effective and essential during such times, because of the need for instant, unquestioned respect for authority and following orders. An army's fight against the enemy in armed combat, a police attempt to control a violent street riot, and the team effort of firemen to control a raging fire while rescuing a family are all examples of the need for unquestioned loyalty to a manager who, by no accident, manytimes has the title of "Commander."

120   Qualities and Strategies of a Good Manager

These are illustrations of crises and emergencies when seconds count and there is no time for a democratic process of calling a time-out in order to ask each soldier, policeman, or fireman for their opinion on the best method for proceeding. The alternative to choosing to obey forced respect is called insubordination, and punishments can range from an army's military court marshal and trial to firing the disobedient member of the police or fire department.

In combat, soldiers tolerate forced respect because they have no choice and they can see valid reasons for the system. In peace time, when there are few valid reasons for the forced system, army officers as well as employees in business and industry will tolerate forced respect only until their patience runs out, and then they quit. In the period of tolerating forced respect, the employee will probably not like her job and therefore not have the interest in producing high quality or quantity work as she might if she enjoyed her work.

> "I really enjoy working for him, because he cares about me...and he often gives me appreciation for my work"

The other type of respect, which is an important part of the positive management approach which we have discussed, is earned respect. To earn the respect of an employee, the employer must first show respect to the employee. This kind of respect results from each party wanting to please the other.

The employer tries to please the employee for 3 primary reasons. First, the employee deserves to be given a humanitarian sense of respect unless they prove that they don't want it or are not deserving of it because of purposeful bad traits. Second, the employee will tend to be happier while performing duties and therefore be more pleasant to have around. Third, the employee will have a greater tendency to like their work and therefore produce a better quality and quantity of work, while desiring to keep their job longer. Think of the PCA as one who "works with you, as an equal in a team," instead of one who "works for you, as a lower subordinate."

The employee, in turn, tries to please the employer for 3 primary reasons. The first 2 reasons are similar to those discussed for employers, in addressing humanitarian respect and the employee's desire to work for a pleasant employer. The third reason addresses keeping the employer pleased so the employer will in turn increase her expressions of appreciation and perhaps salary for work which is done well. As we will see later in this book, that frequent show of appreciation can be much more powerful than occasional salary increases. Employees are willing to work hard in order to receive appreciation.

Or, as Lea, a valued PCA, once told us about the importance of respect from an employer, "I really enjoy working here, because I feel that what I am doing is important. On top of that, I personally feel important because my employer cares about me as a person. I get appreciation for my work and respect for being me. If occasionally he needs something extra done, or my time goes over, I don't mind 'cause I like helping him...often, I actually don't think of it as being work."

By now, you as a reader are probably saying, "OK, you've convinced me to show respect to my PCA and to expect to probably receive it in return. Where do I start? How do I show respect and otherwise begin to practice the positive approach to managing my PCAs?"

There are 4 major components to adopting and maintaining earned respect and the positive approach to management:

a) Your favorable personality and attitude,

b) Your maintaining a pleasant physical work environment,

c) Your routine expressions of appreciation for the PCA and the work he does, and

d) Your consistent respect for the PCA's rights and the practice of other good management techniques.

Each of these 4 major components has many ingredients. Details are found throughout this book.

9. Passive, Aggressive, & Assertive: Which Style is Best for Stating Needs?

There are 3 primary ways that a manager, or anyone, communicates with others: passively, aggressively, or assertively. It is very important that people who make routine requests for assistance from others realize that the clear, direct manner of assertive communication is the best to use, and that they know how to be assertive as well as avoid being weakly passive or abusively aggressive.

It is easy to lose high-quality PCAs by stating your needs in a passive way, and not having your needs heard or understood, or in an aggressive way, and abusing PCAs with requests which are harsh, sarcastic, arrogant, or demanding.

Have you ever heard any of the following comments from others about the way you communicate?:

■ She's so shy...if only she had the courage to speak up for what she needs. (passive)

■ He's so afraid of asking for help and speaking up in a loud enough voice so I can hear him. It's as though he's afraid that I'm going to yell at him or be mad at him for making his needs known. (passive)

■ I wish she weren't so demanding when she asks for help. I'm not her slave. (aggressive)

■ I like the kind of work which I do for him, I just don't like working for him...he's so abusive in the harsh way he demands things! (aggressive)

> Many of us get complaints from PCAs that we are "too demanding"...we often don't understand what PCAs mean or what we can do about it -- here's the answer!

Let's first define and explain each of the 3 communication styles.

A. Passive Behavior

Passive behavior should be avoided since it results in feelings, opinions, and needs which are expressed or only partially expressed in a manner which is weak, poorly understood, or inaudible due to several factors:

1) Weak verbal communication. The speaker either fails completely to express a message or expresses the message in an indirect, incomplete, or implicit manner. An example of a passive statement is: "Gee, the living room sure is getting dusty. I suppose something should be done about it someday," as contrasted with the assertive example of "The living room needs cleaning. Laura, would you please find the time before Friday to vacuum the rug and dust the furniture and window sills."

2) Weak nonverbal communication. The speaker's verbal message is further weakened and confused by poor body language and mannerisms such as avoiding eye contact with the recipient of the message; using a hesitant speech pattern, low voice level, or inappropriate voice tone; mumbling or swallowing words; or making a habit of tense body posture, inappropriate facial expressions, or distracting, nervous gestures.

The negative effects of passive communication are felt by both the speaker and the recipient of messages.

The speaker feels badly about himself because he finds that he is unable to express his opinions or needs. Consequently, his needs are not understood by others and go unfulfilled.

The recipient is unfairly given much of the responsibility for interpreting what message is being sent by the passive speaker. She must spend extra time and energy on figuring out what is being said and questioning the speaker.

B. Aggressive Behavior

Aggressive behavior should also be avoided because it results in feelings, opinions, and needs which are expressed in a manner which is punishing, threatening, assaulting, demanding, or hostile. The rights and feelings of the other individual are not considered and often disregarded or infringed upon. The individual acting aggressively usually assumes little responsibility for the consequences of her actions because she is thinking only about her own needs, feelings, opinions, and objectives during the aggressive communication. Goals are achieved at the expense of other people and obstacles.

Aggressive behavior can be expressed in either a direct or indirect manner, and each manner can consist of verbal or nonverbal communication.

1) Direct verbal aggression. This is characterized by verbal assaults, name calling, threats, or humiliating and hostile remarks. For example, "Look, Tony, I want my breakfast cooked and I want it cooked now. If you don't know how to cook a Johnstown omelette, you must be stupid!"

2) Direct nonverbal aggression. Examples include hostile or threatening gestures, such as fist waving, glaring looks, and "other gestures of the hand," as well as physical assaults.

3) Indirect verbal aggression. Included here are sarcastic comments, catty remarks, and malicious gossip.

4) Indirect nonverbal aggression. This behavior includes physical gestures performed while the intended recipient is not watching, or gestures directed toward objects or toward other people who are not present.

There are negative effects of aggressive behavior for both the speaker and recipient of messages. Each individual feels both short and long term consequences.

The aggressive speaker often receives immediate and more forceful direct counteraggression as a defense from the recipient. This comes in the form of physical and verbal abuse. Indirect counteraggression often comes in the form of a sarcastic reply or defiant glance.

In the long term, aggression often results in strained interpersonal relations. Simply stated, people don't like to be around an abusively aggressive individual. The aggressor may also suffer guilt feelings and regret at having acted aggressively toward others, however he often continues aggressive manners because his goals are realized and therefore the guilt can be overlooked unless excessive. The aggressor often knows of no alternative type of behavior.

For the recipient, or victim of this aggressive behavior, the short-term response can include feelings of humiliation, embarrassment, abuse, resentment, defensiveness, anger, and they may seek revenge by direct or indirect means.

In the long term, the recipient usually wants to avoid as much contact as possible with the aggressor since the contact causes so many negative feelings. As a friend, the recipient will begin avoiding contact and socializing with the aggressor; as an employee, the recipient will begin looking for another job.

C. Assertive behavior

Assertive communication is the desirable way to communicate. It occurs when feelings, opinions, and needs are expressed honestly, clearly, fully, and directly. Others have no need to interpret the message being delivered or the need to defend themselves against abuse, threats, punishments, or other negative feelings of fear and anxiety when assertive communication is used.

> Sometimes we make PCAs mad not because of what we request, but because of the words we choose and the harsh way in which we state the request

Communication is clearly stated, and verbal and nonverbal messages are coordinated and reinforce each other. Also inherent in assertive behavior is a respect for the rights, feelings, problems, and concerns of the recipient of the communication.

It should be recognized that assertive behavior lessens the chance of conflict between two people, but it cannot always prevent conflict. After all, it is the opposing ideas and values which are expressed which cause conflict and not always the way in which they are expressed.

The clear communication of assertive behavior often increases the chances that needs will be understood and that goals will be achieved, but it cannot guarantee such achievements. Regardless of whether goals are realized, the assertive individual realizes satisfaction from succeeding at communicating feelings, opinions, or needs. Regardless of whether the recipient agrees with the communicated message, he appreciates its clear, honest, direct manner and the lack of abuse, anger, and disrespect which come with the aggressive way of speaking.

Assertive behavior produces favorable results for both the speaker and the recipient of the message. These positive results are both short and long term in nature.

For the speaker, initial satisfaction comes from knowing that one's feelings, opinions, and needs have been clearly stated and probably understood. If the the goals behind the communication are achieved, or the recipient agrees with the stated feelings, opinions, or needs, then a second objective is also achieved.

In the long term, routine assertive behavior minimizes the chances of frustrations, depressions, anxiety, and psychosomatic disorders which come with weak, nonassertive communication. It also minimizes chances for the strained relations and guilt which come with aggression. Consequently, relationships with friends and employees will last longer.

For the recipient of spoken messages, the relationship with the individual speaking assertively is usually a comfortable one. This spares the recipient from the fatigue of interpreting and guessing the intention of messages, as occurs with passive communication.

Differences of opinion are certain to occur with any type of communication, but in the long term the recipient usually appreciates the ease of assertive communication. Consequently, the relationship between two individuals will tend to last longer.

In summary, the PCA manager who uses assertive communication will have the satisfaction of clearly making her needs known and increasing the chance that the needs for assistance will be fulfilled. In addition, her PCAs will tend to provide her with better quality work and will need to be replaced less often. This is because her assertive manner shows her respect for them and will make significant contributions to a favorable work environment.

Here are some further illustrations of ways to state needs in 4 situations which are:

(a) assertive (direct, clear, respectful)
(b) passive (weak, incomplete)
(c) aggressive (abusive, hostile, demanding)

1. (a) "Judy, I have a business meeting on Friday morning. Would you mind cleaning my wheelchair by this Thursday night?"

   (b) "My chair is pretty dirty. I hope nobody notices at the Friday meeting."

   (c) "This chair is getting dirty again. I thought we said you'd clean it each week. Let's get it done before Friday or there won't be any Friday paycheck!"

2. (a) "Steve, my shoe is untied. Would you tie it for me?"

   (b) "Gee, shoe's untied."

   (c) "Hey, tie that shoe up, will ya?"

3. (a) "Gillie, before we leave for the shopping mall, would you please put the dishes away?"

   (b) "Could you get to the kitchen sometime?"

   (c) "I don't know why these dishes can't be put away. They've been here all morning."

4. (a) "Cheryl-Lyn, I think I had better use the bathroom before going to bed tonight. Would you mind helping me?"

(b) "I've had a stomach ache all day. Maybe I should use the bathroom sometime."

(c) "I don't know what time you were hoping to leave tonight, but at 8 o'clock I'll need help for an hour in using the bathroom."

5. (a) "Rose, I have noticed the last few mornings that my pant cuffs have been uneven. From now on, would you mind checking them to be sure that they are the same height?"

(b) "My pants sure are looking sloppy lately."

(c) "When I leave for work, I look like a slob because of the lack of caring that you put into this job. Let's be sure those pant cuffs are straight or you and I will have a little talk. Understand?"

10. Job Expectations

A smooth working relationship between an employer and an employee is dependent, in part, on a clear understanding of both the specific job responsibilities and the job expectations.

The "job responsibilities" refer to the list of specific, clear needs for which physical assistance is required. We will discuss the steps in forming this list of needs in a later section of this book.

We will define "job expectations" here as the not-so-clear-but-essential contributions from both the employer and employee toward accomplishing the job responsibilities. These are the factors which are not always stated in the written list of job responsibilities, but which are indeed "expected" to exist if the job is to run smoothly.

> A clear understanding of the job expectations (different from the physical tasks, or "job responsibilities") will help the job run smoothly

To illustrate these, employer contributions can include providing a pleasant work area, giving clear instructions, and paying salaries on a definite schedule. Employee contributions can include maintaining a neat appearance, arriving for work on time, and not stealing personal possessions of the employer.

A clear understanding of both sets of expectations, of you toward the PCA as well as of the PCA toward you, is very important to your success as a manager and consequently to a smoothly running job. These expectations can be put into lists which you can then periodically review to determine whether you are contributing all that you can toward a smooth working relationship. In addition, you may wish to share the following lists with your prospective and hired PCAs, perhaps as a photocopied handout during the interview/screening or the training process.

Here is a partial listing of expectations for both the employer and employee. For each expectation, there is a comparison between the results of both meeting and not meeting the expectation. You will find additional expectations of your own with increased experience as a PCA employer and manager.

A. The PCA's Expectations of You as the Recipient of Services & Perhaps the Employer

Valid Expectations of You

❖ To maintain a clean, reasonably neat personal appearance & to use PCA help as necessary to do so

❖ To keep a clean and bright living space of especially bathroom, bedroom, & kitchen and to use PCA help as necessary to do so

❖ To keep a supply of cleaning aids for you & the PCA to use; for example, disinfectant spray & liquid, spray wax, sponges, paper towels, floor broom-mop-dust pan, bath soap, laundry soap, dish soap, and distilled water for wheelchair batteries

❖ To have a commonsense & efficient layout of your bedroom, bathroom, and other work areas, and therefore to save effort & steps for you and the PCA

Results of Your Failure to Provide this Expectation

❖ To be usually dirty, wear dirty clothes, and smell of sweat, bowel, or urine, and therefore cause PCAs not to want to be near you or work with you

❖ To keep a dirty, dark, and smelly living area with odors of spoiled food, bowel, urine, or dirty laundry and bedding, and therefore to have a poor work environment which PCAs want to avoid

❖ To seldom have a supply of cleaning aids when either routine or unexpected cleaning is required, and therefore to expect the PCA to maintain these supplies or, without supplies, to cause the PCA extra work

❖ To store work items in rooms other than where the items are frequently used, or to store items out-of-reach, and therefore waste time and energy for you and the PCA

Job Expectations

❖ To have a regular order & schedule for doing routine tasks of a daily, weekly, or periodic nature

❖ To have a clear & very complete list of both routine needs & needs which happen occasionally, and to have efficient methods for performing each task ("efficient" = getting the most, high quality work done for the least cost & effort)

❖ To schedule in advance with a PCA most special (nonroutine) projects which are foreseeable, such as defrosting the freezer, cleaning your wheelchair, cleaning windows, or taking clothes to dry cleaners

❖ To ask PCAs in advance if they would mind changing their arrival or departure times or doing something extra

❖ To be assertively clear, direct, and polite in asking or requesting for help from your PCA

❖ To have no logical order or to very often change the order, schedule, and method for doing tasks for no valid reason, and therefore frustrate the PCA whose job is easier when following a routine order

❖ To present new PCAs with an incomplete list of duties, to hide some of your less attractive needs in order to make the job more attractive, & to gradually keep adding duties and therefore frustrate the PCA who sporadically receives new assignments which were not expected

❖ To expect a PCA to often add special projects with no advance request (it is frustrating to run a foot race & have someone unexpectedly move the finish line further away)

❖ To expect on demand and short notice that they will do such special favors, and therefore provide an inconvenience to them

❖ To sharply or sarcastically bark, yell, or snap demands at your PCA in an abusively aggressive way, or to make weak or incomplete requests in a passive style, and therefore to become someone who the PCA tries to avoid

Job Expectations

❖ To assertively keep good eye contact during casual conversations as well as during instructions, compliments, or corrections; good eye contact helps everyone to listen & remember a message (watch actors on TV speak to each other)

❖ To be assertively clear & straightforward in giving a PCA a specific message

❖ To instruct a PCA on how to do a task and then to give him the least supervision necessary, such as only during initial training or when a PCA proves by poor performance that he temporarily needs close, corrective supervision

❖ To welcome suggestions on improving the schedule or methods for doing tasks, even though the employer is not obligated to make changes

❖ To be outwardly happy to see the PCA & welcome the PCA's arrival each time

❖ To passively mumble, speak too softly, and refuse to look at someone while speaking to them resulting in the inability of a PCA to understand my needs

❖ To be "passive aggressive" in giving the PCA merely hints regarding your needs, or being disagreeable & sarcastic with her, hoping she'll "figure out what's wrong or what you need"

❖ To constantly watch, supervise, and correct a PCA who is performing tasks correctly, & to automatically assume that close supervision is always required because PCAs are stupid and not to be trusted

❖ To refuse to even hear suggestions or to tell the PCA to mind his own business, and therefore imply to the PCA that his opinion does not count & is not welcome

❖ To be indifferent, grunt, groan, or show disgust when a PCA arrives, and therefore to cause the PCA to doubt that her work is either important or appreciated

Job Expectations

- To tell the PCA when she is doing a good job

- To politely, firmly, & clearly tell him when he is not doing a good job while explaining why, so he can correct bad habits

- To make a special effort to thank the PCA & show appreciation for the PCA's work each time she leaves

- To pay the PCA promptly on schedule, or to help ensure that 3rd party funding comes on schedule

- To be understanding of the PCA's personal concerns & make reasonable changes in your schedule of needs, as long as your needs are still met and the PCA does not begin to take unfair advantage of your understanding nature

- To be reasonably cheerful & happy and to have a reasonably stable personality

- To not show appreciation when a job is well done, so she doubts that doing a job well is important to you

- To be critical of a bad job without explaining why, and to not provide information on improving job performance

- To be indifferent each time the PCA leaves work, and therefore to give the PCA the impression that her work has not been important & has not been appreciated

- To not care whether the PCA gets a paycheck on time, and therefore cause the PCA anger and frustration

- To be inflexible & not care if the PCA has occasional personal needs or concerns which require you to change your schedule a bit, causing in turn the PCA to not care about your personal needs or concerns

- To have a bad temper, be usually depressed, be a constant complainer, and therefore be someone who is unpleasant to be around

- ❖ To be punctual in meeting the PCA on time, & to contact the PCA in advance if you will be late or absent

- ❖ To have a clear and reasonably organized head

- ❖ To be routinely late to meet the PCA with no advance notice, and therefore to prompt the PCA that he also can be late in meeting your schedule

- ❖ To seldom have a clear head because of abuse of drugs, alcohol, or medications, and therefore to be difficult to work with

B. Your Expectations of the PCA

Your Valid Expectations of the PCA Employee	Results of the PCA's Failure to Provide this Expectation
❖ To be dependable in arriving for work	❖ To not show up at all for work without giving as much advance notice as possible, and therefore forcing you to suddenly - if at all possible - find a replacement at very short notice
❖ To be punctual in arriving for work at the scheduled time	❖ To be routinely late by more than 10 minutes for no valid reason, and therefore either to run out of time before duties are finished or to finish duties but cause both of you to be 10 minutes late in starting the rest of each of your personal schedules
❖ To be dependable in finishing tasks as expected	❖ To leave work with tasks only partially done, and therefore leave you with personal needs unfulfilled
❖ To be responsible for doing routine tasks without constant supervision	❖ To need constant supervision or reminders to do routine tasks, and therefore to cause you unnecessary time & effort
❖ To be responsible for doing tasks in a quality manner with a pride in remembering details	❖ To do tasks with poor quality in a quick manner with little effort or care, and therefore jeopardize your health, safety, or ability to fully function during the day

Job Expectations

❖ To be confidential with your personal concerns, medical needs, beliefs, values, & information about your personal relationships

❖ To be a gossip, backstabber, name caller, or loudmouth who talks with others about your private life

❖ To be honest with your supplies of medications, money, food, and belongings

❖ To "borrow" or steal your possessions, and therefore cost you considerable expense & peace of mind

❖ To respect your intelligence and maturity as someone who is responsible for managing your own needs

❖ To see you as someone who is sick and without abilities, and who is to be pitied and cared for

❖ To want to be a PCA for appropriate reasons of receiving the salary, appreciation for a job well done, a feeling of helping someone, and a straightforward friendship

❖ To want the job for dishonest reasons of wanting my food, money, medications, car, possessions, record/tape collection, sex from you (hetero/homosexual), your boy/girlfriend, a place to hide from police or bill collectors, or someone to hurt, abuse, or control (physically or mentally), & therefore to be an employee to avoid

❖ To appropriately never ask to borrow money from you

❖ To routinely whine & sob for money for various emergencies, and therefore to embarrass you by forcing you to loan money & possibly lose it

❖ To discuss as needed work-related problems for which the PCA desires solutions

❖ To be a constant complainer about problems for which no solutions are proposed or desired

Job Expectations

❖ To keep a neat and clean appearance

❖ To often be dirty in areas of hair, hands, fingernails, or clothes, & to smell of sweat and therefore be an unpleasant employee

❖ To never drink alcohol or take drugs on the job, and to never arrive "under the influence"

❖ To arrive frequently with an alcohol breath or a high from drugs, & therefore endanger your health, safety, or possessions

❖ To listen to your instructions and to do tasks by methods which you have determined are efficient and safe

❖ To ignore your instructions and do tasks the PCA's way, and therefore to cause you to lose your control as an employer in addition to not having your needs met satisfactorily

❖ To offer suggestions to you on improving your schedule or methods for doing tasks

❖ To have no interest in making suggestions, and therefore probably not be interested in performing good quality work

❖ To have the physical, psychological, & emotional abilities to perform the job in a satisfactory manner

❖ To have a physical weakness or emotional instability which interferes with performing expected tasks in a safe, dependable manner

❖ To inform you in advance of crises about work-related problems which are developing and to tell you in advance of any plans to quit

❖ To store up problems until the PCA explodes with anger and possibly quits with no advance notice, and therefore to force you to find a replacement in a hurry

❖ To be honest with you about the schedule & tasks which the PCA is willing to perform, and whether he wants to continue to work for you

❖ To be a chronic liar and give false promises about his willingness to work for you; consequently, he may quit with no advance notice and therefore be someone upon whom you cannot depend

11. The Favorable Physical Work Environment

Regardless of whether you use PCAs from an agency, or you directly employ PCAs and therefore do your own recruiting, interviewing, screening, and training, you will understandably want to keep them as long as possible providing their work is satisfactory. A very important factor in keeping a high quality PCA happy in her job is maintaining a favorable, physical work environment..."a nice place to work."

For a PCA, attractive physical features of a work place include the following:

1) A clean and pleasant work area,

2) An efficient layout of each work area, and

3) A sufficient inventory of the supplies which you need as well as those which the PCA needs.

A Clean and Pleasant Work Area

Few of us would like to live in an area which smells of urine, bowel, or dirty laundry; which has trash overflowing from garbage cans and waste baskets; which has sticky and dirty kitchen counters, table tops, and bathroom sinks and toilets; which has cockroaches or other crawling pests; or which is dark and musty smelling from dirty windows and dusty, drawn shades.

Likewise, few PCAs want to routinely work in such an area, either!

> Providing a pleasant place to work is important to keeping good PCAs happy with their jobs

A clean and pleasant living area for you, and work area for the PCA, does not have to be uncomfortably sterile-clean. Routinely keeping the area clean is not overly time consuming, either. It should have at least the following reasonable features on a regular basis:

a) Not even the slightest trace of smell or odor from urine, bowel, dirty laundry, mold, mildew, or dirty kitchen or refrigerator,

b) All trash, wastepaper, or food garbage kept in wastebaskets or covered trash cans which are kept clean and lined with a plastic bag. The contents are promptly sealed in a tied plastic bag and then disposed of whenever trash either begins to smell or overflow from containers,

c) Clean kitchen countertops, stove areas, and refrigerator interiors. Spoiled food anywhere in the kitchen or refrigerator/freezer areas should be promptly disposed of. After all, "if you can no longer or don't want to eat it, why save it?...throw it out,"

d) Bathroom sinks, toilets, bath/shower, floors, and mirrors cleaned at least once a week,

e) Bed linens changed and all laundry done either promptly after "accidents" or at least once a week,

f) The overall living area should be dusted, vacuumed or mopped, and aired out regularly, and

g) Personal living items should be reasonably organized and neatly stored, as opposed to living among "piles of junk" throughout various rooms.

While it remains your responsibility to provide the PCA and yourself with a clean and pleasant area, the actual physical work (or parts of it) might be beyond your own physical abilities. If so, it is then your responsibility to instruct the PCA in methods and a routine schedule for keeping the area clean. In addition, you are responsible for stocking an adequate variety and quantity of cleaning supplies so that the PCA can do his work. Tips on keeping adequate stocks of supplies, and not running out, are provided later in this section of the text.

An Efficient Layout of Each Work Area

Picture yourself with the job of making hamburgers at a fast food restaurant. Your main work area is a cooking grill and an adjacent table for putting together and wrapping the burgers. Each meat patty is taken from a freezer and cooked on the grill. Then it's placed on a bun and given ketchup, mustard, onions, and 2 pickle slices before the top bun is put into place. You then wrap each burger in paper and place it on a chute where it travels to the customer serving area.

This is really a simple process and should take very little effort. However, suppose each of the ingredients is kept in a different part of the kitchen. You fry (or flame broil!) each patty, walk ten feet to where the buns are piled, walk three feet in the other direction for the ketchup container, reach under the counter for the mustard, and go to the refrigerator for the onions and pickles. After making just your third hamburger, you would probably turn to your boss and say, "Hold it, why can't I organize all of these items around the grill within my reach...this current system is a waste of my energy and time, and therefore wastes a lot of the hourly salary which you are paying me." In the back of your mind you are also telling yourself, "This setup doesn't make sense and it's difficult to work in...if my boss refuses to make it more efficient, then I'll quit and work somewhere else where the work is easier to perform."

Fast food restaurants and all other businesses carefully plan and lay out their various work areas to make them as efficient as possible for employees. So should you for PCAs.

The advantages of efficient work areas for PCAs include saving them energy and time. The PCA can perform his duties much more easily with far less frustration, and therefore you will tend to keep good PCAs longer. Advantages to you include keeping good PCAs longer as well as getting more duties performed during a period of time.

Steps to planning efficient PCA work areas include the following:

1) Identify each work area, or separate location, where the PCA performs a specific set of duties for you: kitchen, bathroom, bedside, dressing area, eating area, etc.

2) For each identified work area, first list the specific set of duties to be performed there and then list the equipment, supplies, articles of your clothing, food, and so forth which the PCA needs for the set of duties in that particular work area. For example, at your bedside work area in the morning the PCA might help you get dressed, and this might require your urinary leg bag, socks, abdominal binder, pants, and belt.

3) Determine the primary one or two places where the PCA actually stands while performing duties within each work area.

4) Design standard locations within the PCA's reach for storing the equipment, supplies, and clothes within each work area. For example, a shelf, drawer, closet, cabinet, pantry, footlocker, shoebox, etc.

> A work area with an efficient layout saves the PCA effort & time

5) Routinely encourage the PCA to keep an organized arrangement of these supplies within each storage area and to return items to their storage place promptly after each time the duties are performed.

A Sufficient Inventory of Supplies

Many of us are quite dependent on a daily or routine use of prescription medications, over the counter medical supplies, and specially prescribed medical appliances and equipment. In addition to personal supplies for our own needs, other types of supplies are required by the PCAs whom we employ. Examples of items they require can include cleaning supplies or tools for assisting in the repair of our medical equipment.

Whether an item is used by you or the PCA who helps you, exhausting your supply of an item can result in one of two situations: a considerable inconvenience or, in fact, a health or life threatening circumstance. This section of the text will provide you with strategies for minimizing the chances of running out of any important supplies.

There is little reason to completely run out of most items. All that is required is some organization and a periodic check on supply levels. There is no additional cost to keeping adequate levels of supplies. "It costs no more to always keep a car's gas tank at least half full, than it does to allow the tank to reach 'empty' before each filling." The overall cost is exactly the same, since the same amount of gas is used in either case...so why frequently gamble on running out?

Keeping an adequate inventory of supplies depends on being able to periodically compare the **actual quantity** of each item that you have stored with the **minimum quantity** needed to prevent running out. For example, if you find that you have a 2-week supply of a medication left, and you believe that it will take 2 weeks to order and receive a new quantity of that medication, then it is now time to reorder.

This periodic comparison of "how much I have" with "the minimum supply needed to get me through reordering" is dependent upon 2 factors. First, since you -- alone -- are always responsible for keeping an adequate supply of each item, the physical storage location of your supplies should be within your personal level of sight (or touch, in the case of a significant sight impairment). In living areas with really limited storage space where not everything can be located at your level of sight or touch, store the least frequently used items where a PCA can periodically check quantities for you at your request.

Second, the arrangement of items within these storage areas should be well organized. A reasonably neat arrangement of items enables you to do two things: to quickly count up the actual quantities of items for inventory purposes, and to quickly locate a specific item whenever it is needed in a hurry. In addition, when you are in a hurry, well-organized items can be easily located by a PCA who is helping you.

This arrangement of stored supplies should take into consideration the following points:

a) Store each type of item together, so that you can determine how many containers of the same item are stocked ahead. For example, store all bottles of medical adhesive together in one section and all boxes of bandages together in another section.

b) When storing each type of item together, reasonably neat rows or sections within a drawer, box, closet, or footlocker will make counting stock much easier than if similar containers are merely tossed into a pile within a box in the back of the closet.

c) Use the entire contents of one container of an item before opening a new container. It is much easier to take inventory if all containers of an item, such as pills, are known to be full except for the one presently being used.

d) In using each container completely before proceeding to the next, it is wise to use the oldest stock first. To make "rotating the stock" easier, many folks write the purchase date on containers of supplies on the day the purchase is made and the container is stored. The PCA then can easily find the next oldest container at your request.

e) To make reordering items easy, keep an index card or computer listing for each type of supply. List the name of the item, the manufacturer, model number, size, and name and phone number of the local store where the item is available. You may wish to include the length of time typically necessary for reordering the item. For example, Urocare urinary leg bag, 1 liter size, # 9032, $28.50 from Wyman's Drug Store, 853-6969; reorder time is usually 2 weeks.

f) When requesting prescriptions for ongoing medications from your physician, ask the doctor if each prescription can be written for at least a month's quantity for each refill, and that each prescription be refillable several times. This strategy can save you extra trips to the pharmacy and to your doctor.

g) The medical supply and equipment business is constantly making improvements in their products. Keep your eyes open at pharmacies and medical supply stores for new or improved supplies which appear on store shelves and in catalogs.

How much of each item you should keep ahead varies for different types of items. To determine what is a "reasonable advance supply," consider the following factors:

a) How often an item is routinely or typically used,

b) What quantity of the item is used each time,

c) Whether an item can be stored ahead without deteriorating, that is whether it has a good shelf or refrigerator life,

d) Whether the item is readily available, for a cash purchase, over the counter (OTC) of a nearby store, or whether its availability is usually delayed by any of the following requirements:

> i) Obtaining or renewing a physician's prescription before being reordered,
>
> ii) Special ordering at a nearby store which does not routinely stock the item on its shelves,
>
> iii) Approval and requisitioning through a funding source (health care plan, insurance company, state or federal program).

> It is your responsibility, and not the PCA's, to keep adequate levels of supplies to prevent "running out" of items

If delays can be expected, determine how much total delay is typical. For planning purposes, double or triple the expected delay estimate to determine how far ahead to order an item. For example, if your physician takes a week to get a prescription renewal to you, a pharmacist then usually requires a week to special order an item, and then Medicaid typically requires a week to process the funding request for you to hand to the pharmacist, then the total typical delay in reordering that item is 3 weeks. To be safe, begin this reordering process at least 6 weeks before your existing supply of the item is due to run out. The extra time allows for "unexpected delays" which can include a physician's unavailability during her vacation, the physician's secretary forgetting to promptly mail you the prescription, the pharmacist forgetting to promptly order the item, the medical supply company's inability to promptly send the order to the pharmacist, Medicaid's backup of paperwork which results in an extra 2 week delay in approval for funding, or the occurrence of a 3-day holiday for everyone during this time.

For many other types of items, obtaining fresh supplies are affected only by one's ability to get to a store. These are the common, over-the-counter (OTC), non-prescription medical products (rubbing alcohol, bandages, aspirin and acetaminophen), personal grooming aids (toothpaste, after shave, feminine hygiene products), and household cleaning items (spray disinfectant and furniture wax, paper towels, plastic trash bags). These are items which are available on store shelves and are usually paid for in cash.

Decisions regarding when to advance stock these "no delay items" depend again upon how frequently each item is used and how much of an item is used each time. Advance stocking of routinely used items does not require a spacious warehouse with a forklift, but actually very little space in your living area. Stocking a bit ahead on a regular basis gives you the advantage of seldom running out of an item at an inconvenient time. In addition, it allows you to buy many items when prices are discounted by sales at local stores and by the manufacturer's discount coupons found in newspapers.

Prescribed Medical Equipment:
Stocking the Supplies & Tools of Preventative Maintenance

Many of us are dependent upon specialized, expensive medical equipment for our mobility, vital body functions, and otherwise staying active and preventing illness or poor health. It is very important to keep an adequate stock of repair supplies and tools. This enables us, or a PCA, to perform preventative maintenance, which prevents many breakdowns from occurring, as well as to perform actual repairs, when unavoidable breakdowns do occur.

The Favorable Physical Work Environment   147

Most of us keep track each day of the weather forecast. After all, we are quite dependent upon the weather when we decide whether to plan an outside activity and, if so, what protective clothing to wear. We have learned that it is often unwise to completely ignore weather forecasts because we might get caught quite unprepared in hot or cold extremes in temperature or in a sudden rain or snow storm. If we haven't heard the forecast, we still pay attention to nature's early warning signs, such as the approach of dark clouds and the rumble of thunder. If we are outside, we take these warning signs seriously and start to protect ourselves from getting soaking wet from the rain or from being hit by lightning.

> How far ahead should you reorder an item? -- Predict when you will run out of an item and decide how long it will take to reorder and receive a new supply, and then double your time estimate to prepare for unforeseeable delays

Preventative maintenance toward the medical equipment upon which we depend is similar to watching the weather, and just as wise. Breakdowns in our equipment are certain to happen, however our preventative maintenance can have 2 advantages. First, routinely taking care of our equipment will prevent some needless breakdowns which might occur from neglect. Second, when an unpreventable breakdown or wearing out of equipment is due to occur, a close familiarity with how that equipment should usually function will manytimes give us some advance warning signs of the upcoming breakdown.

Much like watching for signs of upcoming weather, these warning signs can include an early notice of equipment squeaking or making a strange noise, operating with slowness or difficulty, giving off a strange smell or odor, or, in fact, a flashing or beeping of an equipment's formal warning system. These warning signs are nature's way of telling you of upcoming problems. Be tuned into early warnings, be grateful for them, don't ignore them, and take appropriate action to promptly remedy the problem before the equipment "dies" completely.

If we know in advance that a breakdown is likely to occur we can start in advance on getting the problem repaired, and thus perhaps prevent some breakdowns from even happening. Much like watching the weather, if this advance repair isn't possible we can at least be cautious in our activity to minimize the inconveniences or perhaps dangers of the upcoming breakdown. If we purposely ignore all early warning signs, then we must accept the full consequences of wherever and whenever the equipment suddenly stops operating, and perhaps have to do without it for a considerable length of time while parts are ordered and repairs are made.

Some equipment exams and repairs require professionals. Most professional help is not available immediately and must be arranged in advance through an appointment. Additional delay often occurs -- before the repair appointment can be made -- when the repair will be funded by a third party source and approval for the repair must be obtained in advance. We've heard of one locale where a 3-week approval procedure is required by Medicaid before a simple flat tire on a wheelchair can be fixed at a repair shop; if the repair is made before Medicaid grants their approval, then Medicaid will not fund the repair! As you first acquire a new piece of medical equipment, do some research in advance regarding several places where it can be repaired, whether parts are readily available or must usually be ordered, whether loaner equipment is available while parts are being ordered and repairs are made, and what paperwork and time is required by any funding source which you must use.

Some other equipment exams and repairs can be made by you, possibly with physical assistance from a PCA who follows your instructions. Avoiding the need for professional repair help by "doing it yourself" whenever possible, means a quicker repair without many of the delays and paperwork headaches mentioned above.

> Most unwanted, sudden equipment breakdowns can be prevented from happening by routine preventative maintenance

The Favorable Physical Work Environment 149

Become very familiar with each piece of medical equipment you use. Learn how to spot early warning signs of upcoming breakdowns and act quickly to remedy the problem. Learn, yourself, how to make basic repairs even if you have no physical ability to perform them. If you need physical assistance, then learn how to instruct an available PCA -- step-by-step -- in making those repairs. Do not expect a typical PCA, who doesn't use your medical equipment, to know how to repair it...that's your responsibility.

In speaking of repair supplies, it is also your responsibility to keep an advance supply of those items which you know will probably break down and which are of reasonable cost. If you are unsure of what parts of your equipment will most likely break down or wear out, ask the dealer from whom you purchased the equipment or a professional repairman. Keep an extra of each part which is of reasonable cost and which is easily repaired by you. Such parts can include certain nuts, bolts, tires, tubes, fuses, cane and crutch rubber tips, and wheelchair drive belts.

> When you are outdoors, you watch the sky for warning signs of bad weather; when you use medical equipment, you should watch and listen for warning signs that a part is wearing out -- and get it fixed before it breaks down

To make these repairs, be sure you have an adequate supply of tools which are kept in a locked tool box so that no one "borrows" them. Any lockable area to which PCAs will have periodic access with your permission should be locked with a key, which you keep with you, and not locked with a combination lock. With a key lock, the PCA has access only when you momentarily give her the key; be sure she promptly returns it to you. If you give a PCA the numbered combination to a lock, the PCA can then access the lock whenever she wishes...perhaps without your knowledge.

Purchase good quality screwdrivers (several sizes, regular and phillip heads), pliers, combination wrenches, adjustable wrenches (one large, one small), allen wrenches (one set on a ring or in a jack knife-type casing), tire irons, and a bicycle pump (with a built-in pressure guage). One set of good quality tools, such as those frequently on sale at Sears, is considerably less expensive than buying two or three sets of cheap tools which must be replaced with each tool that bends or breaks. We know...we learned this lesson the expensive way!

One final word on prescribed medical equipment. Each piece of medical equipment which you regularly use will eventually wear out, nomatter how well you maintain it. Learn to recognize, in advance, the time when a piece of equipment is about to wear out and order a replacement. How much in advance? Our previous rule-of-thumb says "two or three times as long as you think necessary to acquire the funding approval, to place the equipment order, and to receive the new item." There are 3 primary ways to estimate the order and delivery time on a piece of equipment:

a) Get a time estimate from each party involved in the ordering process with regard to how long each of their individual involvements will take -- physician, therapist, funding source, pharmacist, medical store, etc., or

> When you receive new equipment, have the basic functions of the old equipment repaired right away so that you will have a readily available backup when your new equipment needs repair

b) Ask a friend, who has ordered and received similar equipment, with regard to the length of the entire process, or

c) Provide your own estimate of time based on your experience in ordering and receiving similar equipment.

If your current wheelchair will soon need replacing, and you believe it will take a 3 month process to receive a new one, then speak up and start the replacement process at least 6 to 9 months before you expect the old wheelchair to become unusable.

After you receive your new chair and you're sure it is working smoothly, give strong consideration to getting the old chair repaired for ready use as a backup to your new chair. The objective is not to replace each old part until the

The Favorable Physical Work Environment

old chair looks like a new one, but instead to repair or replace the few parts which are most worn out and most likely to break down. Consequently, the older wheelchair can be used for brief periods of time when the new chair must be away for either periodic preventative maintenance or unexpected repairs.

Section III

Identifying & Dividing My Needs for Assistance

12) Abusing Help with Inappropriate Requests

13) Types of Activities Which Qualify for PCA Help

14) Making A Master List of Your Needs for Assistance

15) Dividing Needs with More Than One PCA

12. Abusing PCA Help with Inappropriate Requests

Picture yourself in a family in which each member has a set of routine chores for contributing to the smooth running of the family as a whole. Some wash and dry dishes on different nights, another puts out the garbage once a week, another helps with the laundry, and others chip-in parts of their paychecks to the family budget. If all members but one are faithfully making their contributions as agreed, then any lazy member will soon feel quite out-of-place and guilty...and the other members will begin to resent the lack of responsibility of the lazy member not "doing his share."

It is very easy to abuse PCA help by using it to accomplish activities which we could be doing for ourselves. When PCA help is abused,

1) The PCA resents many of the requests for assistance and might lose interest in the job, and

2) We begin to lose respect for ourselves as well as lose some valuable independence.

> Abusing PCA help with inappropriate requests has negative consequences both for the PCA and for you

Like the family members who become upset at the one who doesn't do his share, the PCA can also feel taken advantage of.

When PCA help is abused, the PCA soon begins to wonder why certain requests for help are being made. The PCA was told that she was hired to physically perform activities which the service recipient cannot perform. Consequently, the PCA looks forward to receiving reward both from receiving a salary and from helping someone with activities which they could not experience otherwise. If helping someone toward their own independence were not important to the PCA, then the PCA might instead choose to work as a butler, servant, gardener, or maid. When requests are made for other types of assistance or activities, the PCA begins to feel that she is both not essential and that her assistance is being abused and taken advantage of with

156 Abusing PCA Help with Inappropriate Requests

needless requests. The PCA should feel that she is glad to provide help because the service recipient is doing all that he can for himself. When the PCA is asked to do more than the share for which she was hired, resentment starts to build and she may consequently lose interest in the job.

You, as the service recipient, will also feel negative effects when your PCA help is abused. You may often feel awkward or guilty in not doing your own full share. Second, you will realize that you are gradually losing your ability to live an important portion of your life with independence...the ability to physically do all that you can for yourself, and to manage physical assistance from others for other, appropriate activities.

For many service recipients, this abuse of PCA help -- and the consequent increase of dependence on that help -- is quite similar to an alcohol or drug addiction. The initial habit is easy to acquire and results partially from rejecting rightful responsibilities. The habit grows steadily until the victim begins to feel guilty and a loss of self respect for "refusing to pull one's own weight." At the same time, those around him often begin to resent his lazy and irresponsible behavior. As a result of feeling this "double whammy" from inside and outside, the victim might even slide into a deep depression.

Deciding when it is OK to request help is not as difficult as it may seem. There are distinct categories of needs which do qualify for requesting assistance. These are listed in the next chapter, "Types of Activities Which Qualify for PCA Help."

13. 3 Types of Activities Which Qualify for PCA Help

To prevent abusing PCA help, it is very important that you request --

1) The appropriate type of assistance, and that

2) It is assistance for an appropriate type of activity or need.

Request Primarily Physical Assistance

First, the primary type of assistance requested should be physical assistance. If you are able and willing to manage this help, then you should be performing all of the planning and management duties, especially the following:

a) Listing your needs for assistance from others,

b) Double checking the list to identify any activities which you could be performing for yourself without assistance,

c) Listing the duration, frequency, and schedule for each need to aid your own planning,

> There are 3 main types of needs for which requesting physical assistance from PCAs is acceptable and usually OK

d) Designing the most time-effective and effort-saving methods for a PCA to provide assistance for each need, which in turn enables you to provide clear instructions for the PCA to follow,

e) Performing inventory checks and otherwise maintaining adequate levels of supplies which you and the PCA require, and

f) Otherwise planning, scheduling, and coordinating your own needs with sufficient PCA help.

3 Types of Activities Which Qualify for PCA Help

Second, besides using PCA help primarily for physical assistance, it is important to use assistance only for an appropriate type of activity or need. A need for which you can generally feel comfortable in asking for help will usually be found in one or more of the following categories.

Before citing these 3 categories, it is important to remember that our lifestyle, abilities, health, and stamina do -- indeed -- often change. A physical activity which we can independently perform by ourselves today might temporarily or permanently become a dependent activity tomorrow. Consequently, our need for physical assistance from others will often change...some days will require more, some less.

Here are the categories of situations where you can comfortably ask for assistance:

1) Those activities, or parts of activities, which are truly beyond your own physical abilities,

2) Those activities which, because of physical limitations and not laziness, take too long or use too much personal energy if you attempt to perform them independently, or

3) Those activities which might jeopardize your safety or health if you attempt to perform them independently.

1) Those activities, or parts of activities, which are truly beyond your own physical abilities,

Before you can truly state that you require physical assistance with a particular activity, you must be sure that you cannot perform that activity -- or any part of it -- independently without assistance. In other words, you should feel comfortable and justified in asking for PCA assistance only for those activities which you cannot perform for yourself.

However, for each activity or task which you <u>can</u> do independently for yourself, you should also check the next 2 items in determining whether the task additionally qualifies for assistance from a PCA.

Types of Activities Which Qualify for PCA Help

2) Those activities which, because of physical limitations and not laziness, take too long or use too much personal energy if you attempt to perform them independently,

Many of us have found activities which we can perform independently by ourselves, however experience has shown that independence for this particular task is too costly in terms of the amount of time or energy required of us. For example, some folks have found that they are able to dress themselves each morning. Unfortunately, the time required for this independence might be almost 2 hours, and they are exhausted by the time they are finished. As a remedy, they find that by using PCA help the dressing time is cut to 35 minutes. This savings of time means the ability to get to school or work on time, and with sufficient energy to fully participate in a rigorous daily set of appointments and responsibilities.

The danger presented here to our independence is the easy trap of assigning activities to PCA help for which we are simply too lazy to do for ourselves. There is a fine line between genuinely running short of the time and energy required for meeting schedules and responsibilities, and allowing laziness to tempt us to abuse PCA help with activities for which we have adequate resources but simply lack desire. Remember, abusing PCA help has the serious, negative consequences which we previously discussed.

The objective of using PCA help properly is to conserve time and energy for later use in other schedules of events. Therefore, one may find ironically that increased PCA help is required as one adds more time and energy responsibilities to one's daily lifestyle. In other words, you might now require less PCA help if your current daily schedule and few responsibilities do not require you to be at a full day's school or work by 8:30 each morning. If you acquire such a full day's schedule of responsibilities and appointments in the future, however, you might find that increased PCA help is necessary in such areas as shopping, laundry, housecleaning, cooking, and washing dishes.

In addition to determining whether an activity is beyond our physical limitations or takes too much time and energy, we should ask whether the activity is safe for us to perform on our own.

3) Those activities which might jeopardize your safety or health if you attempt to perform them independently.

In our above example, we illustrate a situation where one lacks the sufficient time or energy for dressing or grooming in the morning. Let's imagine that the attempt to be independent in dressing in bed also routinely resulted in bedsores of the elbows as one repeatedly maneuvered in bed; that poorly positioned support stockings occasionally produced pressure sores on the feet or heels; that one's poor trunk balance during independent bed-to-wheelchair transfers resulted in occasional tumbles onto the floor; or that one's attempt to independently cook certain foods resulted in the risky handling of hot saucepans or pots of boiling water.

In these situations, performing these activities with certain physical limitations and without assistance clearly provides a jeopardy to one's health or safety. When one's health or safety is endangered by independently attempting certain activities, then that unassisted activity is, in fact, counterproductive to independent living. After all, there isn't much feeling of independent living during the many weeks while one is confined to bed while healing a pressure sore or severe burns.

Without safety and health, there is very little independent living. If you cannot perform a task safely, and in a manner which preserves health, then don't allow a false sense of independence and pride to convince you to act foolishly by attempting an activity without assistance. Ask for help and know that you are justified in doing so.

Types of Activities Which Qualify for PCA Help   161

4 Ways to Request Help from PCAs

When you have determined that it is OK to request assistance for a particular need, you will find that the need usually falls into one of 4 situations. Each of these situations requires a different strategy for acquiring PCA help.

It is important to understand each situation type so we can realize the appropriate way to request PCA help in each case. If this does not at first seem to be important, consider the following frequent, classic complaints from PCAs...and how much you would like to avoid them from recurring:

■ "You make too many demands; I'm not a slave."
■ "I need time to myself when I don't feel like I'm 'on-duty' by waiting on you; some of your needs could wait for a time when giving you assistance is more convenient to me."
■ "I don't have time for your unscheduled need; you should have told me in advance so I could have planned enough time."
■ "You shouldn't 'cry wolf' by claiming that a need for assistance is urgent or an emergency, when it isn't and you simply want trivial attention in a hurry!"
■ "This was a real emergency; you should not hesitate to ask for help at times like this!"
■ "Anytime you need anything, you just ask and I'll be glad to help you." (But when you do ask for help, the PCA makes it clear that she is not at all 'glad to help you'!)

Knowing when to ask for help and when your request will be resented by a PCA can be confusing, frustrating, and emotionally upsetting. "Should I ask for help now, or wait for a while?" Details of the following 4 types of situations might help you answer that question in the future.

> Each valid need for PCA assistance usually falls into one of 4 situations, and each situation calls for a different strategy or way for asking for PCA help

I. Needs which can be listed in advance. The first type of situation is one in which the need is foreseeable, usually occurs routinely, and for which the need (and its duration, frequency, logical order, and schedule) can be listed in advance on one's master list and schedule of needs. The steps to creating a master list of needs are discussed in another chapter of this book, "Making a Master List of Your Needs for Assistance."

Examples can include daily dressing and grooming, bi-weekly laundry, weekly shopping, routinely watering house plants, or any predictable and routine need for assistance.

Assistance is appropriately obtained by planning and scheduling PCA help in advance as part of one's routine. These needs should be clearly listed in one's master list, and discussed with the PCA at the time he is hired for the job.

II. Needs which can be scheduled only as each need becomes apparent. The second type of situation is that which is not routine, might or might not be foreseeable, and for which the method and scheduling can be determined only in close advance of, or at the time of, the need.

These can be special one-shot or occasional projects such as cleaning the wheelchair, repairing an almost worn-out wheelchair part, washing apartment windows, or waxing the car.

Assistance is appropriately obtained by requesting PCA help in advance as much as possible, and avoiding last-minute requests whenever possible. At the time the need becomes evident, state the need to the PCA, how soon it should be accomplished, and ask the PCA when (within the stated time period) it would be convenient for her to provide the assistance. In contrast, a common mistake is made when one expects a PCA to suddenly add new duties to today's list, when instead the special duties could be reasonably scheduled in advance for the convenience of the PCA.

> If you know which needs qualify for PCA help, and which strategy to use in asking for that help, then being assertive in making your request will be much easier for you

Types of Activities Which Qualify for PCA Help

As an illustration, Walter decides that he would like to have his wheelchair cleaned this week because he plans to attend his cousin's wedding on Saturday. The following statement illustrates an appropriate, assertive way to request assistance for sporadic needs:

> Walter: "Cheryl-Lyn, my cousin's wedding is this coming Saturday at Shelton Hall in Boston, and I would like my wheelchair cleaned before I attend the wedding. When, during this week, would it be convenient for you to clean it?"

III. Needs which are mere inconveniences. The third type of need is that which is not foreseeable, and which does not require immediate assistance because it merely presents an inconvenience.

Examples can include dropping eye glasses or a book on the floor, noting that a desired book is out-of-reach, having the plug to the TV pull from the wall outlet, or noting that the afternoon sun is bright and wishing that the windowshades were drawn.

Assistance is appropriately obtained by waiting until help is next available, and not by calling specially for help unless the PCA is already in the immediate area.

A common mistake with this kind of need is to label the need as being urgent or an emergency, and consequently demanding help immediately. The PCA soon resents being told, "I want help, I want it now, and it's your job to give me help whenever I want it because you work for me and I sign your paycheck!"

| The rule-of-thumb definition for an emergency is "a situation where the property, safety, or health of anyone is in immediate danger or jeopardy" |

If a need is not urgent, do not label it as urgent. If it is urgent, and the reason might not be obvious, then explain why it is urgent when you receive the help. If you "cry wolf" with false urgencies too often, the PCA will quickly begin to resent your strategy.

Also, attempt to increase your independence by devising ways to remedy similar future situations by yourself. For example, if a desired book is often out of reach when no assistance is available, then try to prevent the same inconvenience in the future by anticipating, in advance, which books you might need and requesting them before the PCA leaves. If your glasses fall onto the floor, then try to design some reaching aid to enable you to pick them up by yourself.

IV. Needs which are true emergencies. The fourth type of need is that which is not foreseeable, can occur with any frequency, and which requires immediate assistance or medical attention because it presents a direct threat to safety, health, or property.

Examples can include the feeling of severe bowel or bladder distention, experiencing the initial stages of falling out of bed, requiring out-of-reach medication for a sudden health concern which is not routine, needing a blanket in the middle of the night, or smelling or seeing smoke in your environment.

Assistance is appropriately obtained, depending on the type and urgency of assistance required, by calling a PCA, neighbor, passer-by, police, fire department, ambulance, etc. If you have carefully and rationally identified a need as being truly urgent or as an emergency, then you are justified in making an appropriately urgent request for help. The rule-of-thumb definition for an emergency is "a situation where property, safety, or health of anyone is in immediate d anger or jeopardy."

14. Making A Master List of Your Needs for Assistance

Before the first PCA can be hired to provide help, you should identify and list the items with which you believe you require help. The time and effort necessary for writing out this master list are similar to those encountered in writing out one's personal resume of education and work experience. The process of establishing the list for the first time can be tedious and time consuming, however the resulting product serves several important purposes listed below. Once the initial list has been completed, making periodic, updated revisions is much easier especially if the list is stored on a computer.

Advantages to Making a List

The advantages of making this master list of routine and nonroutine needs include the following:

a) To help you realize the details and schedule for each foreseeable activity, for which you request physical assistance from someone else, so that you can more easily plan in advance to have PCA help each time you need it,

> Just as a building contractor requires a blueprint in order to instruct construction help, you should write out a master list of your own needs before instructing PCA help

Our overall goal of managing PCA help is to match our needs for physical assistance with the physical assistance available from PCAs. It is common sense logic that we -- as service recipients -- must know the specific needs for which we require assistance before we will be able to hire PCAs to provide that assistance. In the same way, an architect who wants to construct a building cannot logically hire a construction crew and order the delivery of construction materials before he has first drawn up detailed blueprints which make possible providing instruction to the crews.

166   Making A Master List of Your Needs for Assistance

b) To enable you to periodically review the list to determine whether the list of needs and schedule has changed and needs updating because your lifestyle has changed,

> For most of us, life brings a steady stream of changes since, as the saying goes "nothing stays the same for very long." This means changes in where we live, with whom we live, our medical situation, our abilities and stamina, and our daily responsibilities and consequent schedule. With many of these changes come changes in our requirements for assistance from others. Once a master list of needs has been compiled, periodically updating that list is easy. The alternative to keeping an updated written list is to attempt to remember all details of the master list, and juggle changes, in our head. Take advice from the experience of others: the written list is much easier to maintain, visualize, and remember!

c) To enable you to periodically review the list to determine whether you could perform any of those activities independently without assistance from someone else,

> Since each of us is interested in maximizing our personal independence, we should continually try to do more and more for ourselves without assistance from others. The process of learning new rehab techniques does not end with our discharge from a rehabilitation hospital...it is a life-long process which we continue on our own. The written master list of our needs provides an easy way to periodically review the activities for which we believe we need assistance, and to choose certain activities for trying new independence techniques. Whenever we succeed in performing a new activity for ourselves, we can be proud of removing that activity from the written master list of needs for assistance.

d) To enable you to include this list within the PCA job description which each prospective PCA will want to see before knowing whether he wants to work for you. For more details on both creating a job description and using it, see the chapters "Creating a PCA Job Description for PCAs" and "Interviewing,"

> An essential step in hiring new PCAs is to interview prospects. The interview process enables you to

Making A Master List of Your Needs for Assistance

determine whether a prospect is desirable for you to hire. In addition, it enables prospective PCAs to determine whether they can adequately perform the job and want the job. Before prospects can make these determinations, they must know specifically what duties will be expected of them. The most clear method of outlining duties during the interview is to present each prospect with a written job description. The majority of a well written job description is the detail found in the master list of needs. The other types of information to be included in a job description are outlined in a later chapter, "Creating A Job Description for PCAs."

> Your master list should include all of your routine and nonroutine needs; don't cheat by leaving out less attractive or unpleasant needs

e) To enable you to easily visualize the schedule and number of your needs so that you can determine logical ways of dividing your needs among more than one PCA. For more details, see the chapter "Dividing Needs with More Than One PCA."

In that upcoming chapter of this book, information is provided about dividing your needs for physical assistance among more than one PCA. In this later section are reasons why dividing needs might be a good idea for you, as well as strategies for deciding how to logically divide those needs. If you find that dividing needs is a wise management technique for your situation, then compiling this master list of needs is the first step toward that procedure. Without this written master, making decisions about logical and efficient divisions of your needs is considerably more difficult.

Steps to Follow in Making Your List

Steps to follow in creating a master list of routine needs include the following:

1) Write out a list of each activity or need for which you believe you require physical assistance from someone else.

168   Making A Master List of Your Needs for Assistance

In your mind, "walk through" the activities of a routine day from the time you wake up on a typical morning. Write down each activity, or group of activities, for which you usually require physical assistance. You will find it very useful to include the following in a 4-column listing:

a) A brief title or descriptor for each need or logical grouping of needs,

> It isn't necessary to list every single step of the routine for which you require assistance, however you may wish to list the titles of main, primary needs or groups of needs.

b) The approximate duration of time necessary for each need, that is, how long each need requires assistance,

> The approximate durations listed in this next column are intended to provide merely planning guidelines. The objective is not to provide a rigid, minute-by-minute schedule which the PCA must follow.

c) The frequency and schedule for each need, such as by stating one or more of these:

- "x times each (day, week, month, season, year, etc.)"
- "morning, noon, afternoon, evening, etc."
- "each (specified day)"
- "before, after (a specified time of day)"
- "unpredictable" [for those needs which occur without warning or which occur with no predictable schedule]

> This third column of information tells you and the PCA how often a specified need occurs. In addition, it might state the actual days of the week or a similar schedule when a need occurs.

> However, some needs occur on an unpredictable basis. Examples can include the cleanup for bowel or bladder accidents, assistance for the repair of wheelchair or equipment breakdowns, and the extra duties which might be realized when the service recipient becomes sick or develops any special medical problem which requires additional care. These needs for assistance from others are, indeed, foreseeable even though the

Making A Master List of Your Needs for Assistance 169

frequency and schedule for their actual occurrence is unpredictable. You are doing both yourself and the PCAs a disservice to adequate planning if you fail to include these unpredictable needs in your list. Such needs are certain to occur, you just can't predict exactly when they will occur. Be sure to list them.

d) The ideal times, or range of times, for starting and ending the requested help.

Again, these approximate times are not intended to provide a rigid minute-by-minute schedule which limit the flexibility for you and the PCAs. Instead, they are merely guildelines for planning purposes.

2) After you have completed this list from memory, keep it handy and review it for the next several days as you actually ask for assistance for various needs. Check your list to be sure that each actual request is on your list and that the details of each of the 4 columns is accurate.

3) Be sure to list both those activities which occur each day, as well as those which occur less often. Your list should include each foreseeable activity, regardless of whether it occurs each day, two or three times per week, once or twice a month, on a seasonal schedule, or even on an unpredictable frequency and schedule.

4) Next, review the list to determine whether you could perform any of the needs -- or even part of a need -- independently without assistance. If so, practice ways for performing the activity by yourself. If you are successful, then congratulate yourself for a step toward further independence and remove that activity from your list.

5) When you believe your list is complete, compare the items with the previously discussed three categories of activities for which requesting PCA help is appropriate (see the chapter "Types of Activities Which Qualify for PCA Help.") Each of the items on your master list of needs for assistance should be described by one or more of those 3 categories.

Making A Master List of Your Needs for Assistance

An Example
An example of a partial master list of needs, with illustrations of male and female needs, is shown below:

A Master List of Needs for Assistance

Title of Need	How Long	Frequency	Approx Start/Stop Times
▮ morning meds in bed	2 min	each morn	7 am
▮ empty bladder	2 min	each morn	
▮ change urinary device/feminine napkin	10 min	each morn	7:05-7:15
▮ begin dressing in bed: socks, binder, underware	10 min	each morn	7:15-7.25
▮ transfer to wheelchair & adjust position	5 min	each morn	7:25-7:30
▮ wash & groom at sink	20 min	each morn	7:30-7:50
▮ finish dressing from waist up	5 min	each morn	7:50-7:55
▮ cook breakfast, eat, put dishes into d'washer	20 min	each morn	8:00-8:20
▮ dress for outside & transfer to car	10 min	each wkday	8:20-8:30
▮ commute to work with driver	20 min	each wkday	8:30-8:50
▮ at work: transfer from car to wheelchair & go to worksite	10 min	each wkday	8:50-9:00
▮ meet PCA to empty legbag in restroom	10 min	each wkday	10am, 12n, 2pm, 4pm
▮ meet PCA or cafeteria staff for lunchroom help: go thru line, get food, carry tray to table, prepare food, eat	45 min	each wkday	11a-12:30p

Making A Master List of Your Needs for Assistance 171

- meet PCA at home
for lunch: cook,
serve food, eat   45 min   each
                                    nonworkdy 11a-12:30p
- dress for outside
& transfer to car   10 min   each wkday 5-5:10pm
- commute to home
with driver   30 min   each wkday 5:15-5:45
- transfer from car   10 min   each wkday 5:50-6:00
- cook dinner, serve
food, eat, dishes into
d'washer   60 min   each eve   6:00-7:00
- grocery shop   2 hrs   Fri eves   7:15-9:15p
- laundry   3 hrs   M-Th eves &
                                    on day of
                                    accidents   after 7pm

- mop kitchen &
bath floors, vacuum,
bedroom & living
room, clean
bathroom sinks-
mirror-toilet-shower,
change bedsheets   45 min   M-Th eves
                                    during
                                    laundry   after 7pm
- water plants   20 min   M-W-F eves after 7 pm
- bowel/douche
routine & shower   1.5 hrs   Su-T-Th
                                    eves   7:30-9:00p
- help into bed:
wash at sink, eve
meds, transfer to
bed, undress, &
position   25 min   each night 10-10:25p
- bowel or bladder
accident cleanup   1 hr ave   unpredictable
- clean wheelchair,
check battery levels   20 min   once/week   after dinner
- repair wheelchr   varies   unpredictable
- defrost kitchen
freezer   20 min   spring & fall
- wash & wax car   3 hrs   spring & fall
- wash apartment
windows   2 hrs   spring & fall

15. Dividing Needs with More Than One PCA

Many people who employ PCA assistance find several advantages in routinely employing more than one full-time or part-time PCA. The needs for assistance are divided among the PCAs by categories of need, schedule, or by any of several other factors. It is true that there is an arbitrary minimum number of needs for assistance which makes employing more than one PCA impractical, however most people will find a logical way to divide their needs in order to benefit from the advantages of this system.

Advantages to Dividing

There are several advantages to dividing your needs for assistance with more than one PCA.

1) Several PCAs cost no more than just one PCA, and maybe less

2) Reduce the chance for a PCA wanting to quit due to burnout

3) Instant availability of backup PCAs when one PCA is suddenly unable to work

4) Ease your ability to maintain quality control over poor PCA attitude or performance

5) Reduce your reluctance to request assistance from a PCA who has a negative attitude

6) Ease finding assistance for a variety of needs when several PCAs have a variety of skills

1) Several PCAs cost no more than just one PCA, and maybe less

   The strategy of hiring more than one PCA does not mean that you require the financial resources to hire a staff of full time people. On the contrary, the strategy merely means dividing a well written master list of needs among more than one part-time PCA.

For example, if you require PCA help for 28 hours per week, or approximately 4 hours per day, then you might somehow hope to keep one PCA happy while she performs all 28 hours of weekly work, every day, week after week, month after month. Or, for the same cost in salary, you can hire two, three, or more part time PCAs to each work part of that 28-hour week...and you will realize each of the other five benefits outlined below.

> There are several proven advantages to using more than one part-time PCA

In fact, within certain circumstances, you might actually save money and paperwork. In some situations, employing several part-time employees instead of one, full-timer saves the employer from the legal obligations of paying FICA and unemployment taxes and therefore from filing forms and paying certain periodic taxes. This topic is discussed later in this book in the chapter "Tax Obligations for a PCA Employer."

2) Reduce the chance for a PCA wanting to quit due to burnout

Whenever just one PCA is responsible for someone else's entire set of needs, day-after-day without any relief, there is an increased chance that the PCA will prematurely lose interest in the job, become tired of the work, and decide to quit. There are several factors which contribute to this burnout and which can be minimized by spreading one's needs with more than one PCA.

In an overall sense, one PCA working alone has no opportunity for "time off" from the work, and no relief from the constant feeling of the "on duty" responsibility for providing assistance to a very dependent individual.

Your needs for assistance occur day-after-day, week-after-week, and month-after-month with no pauses or holidays. Whether you obtain PCA help from your spouse, relatives, or salaried employees, these people need time off for at least 2 reasons: to provide an "off duty" break from the constant responsibility of the work (and the feeling of your dependence on them) and to provide them the chance to pursue their own interests of career, education, or leisure activities.

Whether a worker performs PCA duties, cooks hamburgers at a fast food restaurant, or buys and sells stocks at an investment brokerage on Wall Street, their mind and body requires routinely scheduled time off. Psychological and sociological studies of workers in many occupations have shown that when workers are forced to work long hours, days, or months without the chance to look forward to regularly scheduled time off, negative psychological and physiological health problems occur -- and workers quit their jobs.

3) Instant availability of backup PCAs when one PCA is suddenly unable to work

An old saying wisely states "Don't put all of your eggs in one basket." For our purposes, we could rephrase this addage to state "Don't put all of your needs for assistance with just one PCA." In the first case, if the bottom suddenly falls out of the one basket, there is no backup protection for your entire collection of eggs; in the second case, if the one PCA is suddenly unable to work, is fired, or quits, there is no backup assistance for your entire set of needs.

> If you "wouldn't put all of your eggs in one basket," why "trust all of your needs with just one PCA"?!

When a PCA can no longer work, there is a sudden need to find a replacement. PCA replacements have to be found for many reasons. Sometimes a PCA is temporarily unable to work due to illness or personal reasons. At other times, a PCA must be fired or decides to quit. There might be a need for a temporary fill-in or a long-term replacement. This help can be found through 5 main sources.

   a) Other PCAs whom you already employ, and who are willing to temporarily fill in a few extra hours until a replacement is found,

b) PCAs you formerly employed, and who are willing to temporarily fill in a few hours until a replacement is found,

c) Friends or relatives who are willing to temporarily fill in a few hours until a replacement is found,

d) Prospective PCAs whom you previously interviewed and kept in your files as a "second priority" and who are willing either to temporarily fill in a few hours until a replacement is found or to be hired as the replacement, and

e) A new PCA prospect whom you recruit, interview, screen, and train from scratch as the replacement.

These 5 sources and others will be discussed in more detail in the chapter of this book entitled "Sources for Recruiting PCAs," however we should note at this time that the most easily tapped source for temporary fill-ins is using extra hours from other, already employed PCAs until a replacement is found. These are the other PCAs who already work for you, know your routine, and who are usually willing to each assume a few extra hours of salaried help until either the temporarily incapacitated PCA returns to work or a new PCA replacement is hired.

4) Ease your ability to maintain quality control over poor PCA attitude or performance

When you are dependent upon just one PCA for providing assistance for all of your needs, there is a natural fear in losing that only source of assistance if the PCA becomes unhappy with her work. To keep the PCA happy, there is an understandable reluctance to correct most poor attitude or work performance problems of the PCA. In such a "one PCA town," you can easily fear that if the PCA becomes offended or mad, she will quit and you will have no assistance for an unpredictable period of time until you can find a temporary fill in or longer-term replacement.

There are unavoidable circumstances between every employer and worker when the employer must discuss worker attitude or performance problems which are occurring. If the employer feels that these discussions about quality control cannot take place, then the employer has lost management control of the work situation. When the employer loses his control, the quality of work as well as the employer-worker relationship have a probable chance of steadily decreasing until the worker usually quits. This occurs because the worker gains increasing control, steadily loses respect for the employer, and takes more and more unfair advantage of the employer and the situation.

Every employer must safeguard their right to constantly maintain quality control by whatever means are necessary, including usually first attempting to correct worker behavior and then, if necessary, firing the worker.

When you divide duties with more than one PCA, and the other PCAs can together provide an instant, temporary fill-in for any one PCA, then you, the employer, are in a much better position to discuss unpopular topics with any employee. In turn, when an employee knows that she can be quickly replaced if her attitude or work is not satisfactory, then she knows that she can lose her job and therefore has an incentive to correct her behavior. In contrast, if the employee knows that a replacement would not be easily possible, then the employee knows that she is in control and has little incentive to correct poor behavior.

5) Reduce your reluctance to request assistance from a PCA who has a negative attitude

When there is only one PCA to provide assistance, and that PCA has a negative attitude toward you or your needs, then you will have a natural reluctance to request any assistance which might offend the PCA and therefore increase the negative attitude toward you. As in our previous discussion about an understandable fear to assert one's right to quality control, this similar fear to request assistance also comes from the concern of losing one's only source of help. Unscrupulous PCAs quickly recognize this fear and take unfair advantage of their very powerful opportunity to "bully around" and even mistreat the employer who depends on them. Once more, the employee has taken control of the employment situation...and the quality of assistance will steadily decrease until the PCA usually decides to suddenly quit.

What you, the victim, in such an unpleasant situation want to do is to fire the negative PCA and replace her with someone with a positive attitude. When you employ more than one PCA, the chances are good that you can do so.

When more than one PCA is employed, it is easier for you to be assertive and ask for help. With more than one PCA, each employee realizes that she is replaceable, can lose her job, and therefore has an incentive to respect the employer, provide quality work, and avoid negative attitudes.

6) Ease finding assistance for a variety of needs when several PCAs have a variety of skills

Many of us require assistance for several types of needs. The variety of types can include the wide range of medical needs, household cleaning, mechanical repairs to mobility equipment and household furnishings, yardwork around the house, and transportation driving. It would be rare to find one PCA who, alone, is skilled and willing to perform this complete variety of needs.

By hiring more than one PCA, one is hiring a wider range of skills and increasing the chances that assistance will be available for a wider variety of needs. In addition, when specific PCA skills are matched with specific types of needs, the recipient of services receives a higher quality of help.

When Dividing Duties is Wise & Unwise

There are 6 primary factors, any one of which indicates that employing more than one PCA might be a wise strategy:

1) If you often need assistance for several hours, either in straight shifts or in separated blocks of time,

2) If you need assistance several days per week,

3) If you need assistance at more than one location,

4) If you need a variety of types of help,

5) If you find that people in your area who are willing to perform PCA duties are available only for part time work which comes in small blocks of time, or

6) If you find that people in your area who are willing to perform PCA duties have a strong tendency to change jobs often, and therefore you have a frequent turnover in the PCAs whom you hire.

> There are 2 primary situations where dividing your needs just isn't possible

There are some situations when employing more than one PCA is not practical. These situations include the following:

1) If you have very few needs for assistance, and there are too few needs for the routine employment of more than one PCA,

> Some folks need very little assistance. Examples might include someone needing help only with a 1 1/2 hour bowel or douche program and shower on 3 evenings per week, or one 3-hour period each week of doing laundry, assisting with grocery shopping, or performing housecleaning. In these circumstances, a PCA would probably be unwilling to come to work for you for any shorter period of time, and therefore dividing a single duty would not be practical. If in the future the individual in any such single-duty circumstance finds the need to add duties at other scheduled times, then the 2nd PCA could be hired instead of merely offering the additional duties to the first PCA.

> There are 6 main strategies for deciding how to divide your needs

2) If you receive 3rd party funding for PCAs, or receive PCAs through a nursing or home health agency who employs them for you, and the funding or agency policies restrict you from using more than one PCA.

Dividing Needs with More Than One PCA

These are unfortunate circumstances when an employing agency or funding source is unwilling to provide or fund more than one PCA because "it doesn't seem necessary"...in reality, they are saying that they are unwilling to put effort into additional recruiting and paperwork. As we have discussed, dividing duties does not bring additional salary expense. Ironically, many agencies are unable to readily provide fill-ins when a regularly scheduled home health aide is unable to work. This situation could be partially remedied if they employed more, part-time staff and avoided "putting all (of your) needs for assistance in one PCA."

Strategies for Dividing Your Needs

If you decide to consider dividing your needs, there are 6 primary factors for deciding how to divide your needs among more than one PCA:

1) Time of day; for example , assign morning needs to 1 PCA and evening needs to another,

2) Days of the week; for example, assign M-W-F needs to 1 PCA and T-Th needs to another,

3) Weekends; for example, assign weekend needs to 1 PCA, or to different PCAs on different weekends on a rotating monthly schedule,

4) Location; for example, assign home needs to 1 PCA and work/school needs to another,

5) Types of work; for example, divide different types of needs among different part-time PCAs who have various skills and interests -- medical assistance, household cleaning, mechanical repairs of mobility equipment and household furnishings, yardwork, transportation driving, or

6) Amount of work; for example, if 2 or 3 PCAs can each work for only limited blocks of hours, divide your total schedule of needs accordingly among all 3 PCAs, instead of trying to find one PCA to fulfill all of your needs.

180   Dividing Needs with More Than One PCA

The managerial process is simple for actually dividing your needs among more than one PCA, or for developing any type of PCA work schedule. Since planning of any kind is one of your responsibilities, and PCAs should provide only physical assistance, it is your job to decide how the schedule of your needs should be divided and then to implement that schedule with the PCAs.

You will require two basic kinds of planning information:

a) Your master list and schedule of needs for assistance, and

b) The list of the PCAs and the schedule of days and times that each is available to work.

The process is for you to draw up a PCA work schedule by matching your schedule of needs with their available times. After you have decided how you believe the divisions should occur, some situations allow you to simply tell the PCAs of their assignments while inviting feedback. This strategy can be used where the different PCAs are performing different types of work, and they are not working closely together. In other situations, where PCAs work closely together and do similar tasks, you may wish to make a photocopy of the matchup schedule for each PCA, call them together in a meeting, and ask for their reactions and advice to your proposed schedule.

Remember that by putting the PCAs in an advisory capacity, you -- the manager -- still retain all final decisions. However, be ready to make reasonable compromises. It is quite important to make the PCAs advisors to the decision-making process, so that they know that their opinion counts. Otherwise, they will feel that they are "being told" what schedule to work.

Listen openly to the concerns and preferences which the PCAs voice, and make any changes which seem appropriate...changes both which make the PCAs happier and which do not sacrifice important details of your needs. Some managers ignore the opinions and preferences of their employees, while believing that seeking employee advice is a sign of a weak manager. On the contrary, it is the strong managers who seek employee advice and who keep employees happier in that way. More details about managerial strategies are found in the chapter "Qualities and Strategies of a Good Manager."

In addition to this set of initial decisions leading to a PCA work schedule, you should clearly state that the PCAs should feel free to discuss among themselves and with you any desired future changes in the schedule which they wish to make. Encourage them to discuss the exchanges of duty times among themselves, and then to bring their proposals to you for approval. The alternative is for each PCA to simply notify you of schedule problems, and for you to be entirely responsible for contacting each of the other PCAs to create solutions. Instead, save yourself for the approval stage by requiring PCAs to find their own solutions to desired work and schedule changes and exchanges.

Section IV

Paying Salaries & Taxes

16) Methods for Paying PCAs

17) Salaries: Determining Salary Rates & Merit Increases

18) Monetary Salaries: Cash, Noncash, or Both

19) U.S. Tax Obligations for a PCA Employer

20) Medical Deductions & Credits for PCA Employers (U.S.)

21) A Listing of U.S. Tax Publications for PCA Employers

16. Methods for Paying PCAs

Volunteer PCA Help: Don't Over-Use It or Rely on It

First, should I use volunteers? The temptation to try to use volunteers is a strong one, especially if paying a salary to a PCA would come from one's personal finances. After all, the monetary savings would be considerable and there would be no tax forms to file or taxes to pay.

Additionally, some folks routinely and very successfully use volunteer help from agencies which recruit and maintain large pools of volunteers. Examples include people who wish to perform volunteer reading, tutoring, and companionship to leisure and shopping events.

However, for any recurring or extensive PCA need for which you are very dependent upon personal medical assistance, volunteer help is definitely not the answer. Problems too often happen with the length, punctuality, and dependability of their assistance for PCA needs. Nevertheless, volunteer help is sometimes adequate for brief, one-shot needs for assistance. In other words, for brief needs, don't over-use it, and for needs in general, don't rely on it. Consider the following common experience.

> Many of us have lived for a time in a college campus dormitory or residence hall. We occupied one of the 75 two-man rooms in the dorm, and became friends with many of the other 150 students who also lived in the same building. Several of these folks often told us, especially when they first met us at the beginning of each new year, "Hey, if you ever need any help, don't hesitate to ask...I'll be glad to do you a favor anytime."

> Routinely expressing appreciation for good-quality work is a very powerful way to keep a good PCA happy with her job

> For an occasional, one-shot, brief need, these good buddies were usually willing to help out...if they were not already busy in their own academic study or another

activity. However, some of us soon wore out our Good Samaritan welcome by asking for favors too frequently.

We would drop a book on the floor in our room, the typewriter wasn't plugged in when we wanted to type a report, or our leg bag needed an empty before the salaried PCA was scheduled to return. Some of us also had come to the large campus with a manual wheelchair when our limited ability really required a motorized wheelchair. Our personal pride had clouded over reality and we had refused the suggestion of getting something motorized. As a consequence, some of us were always begging for a push to class, a push to the library, or a push to the pizza place downtown. It wasn't long before our fellow residents just didn't seem as friendly toward us as they used to be.

Oh, no one ever outwardly complained, and when we asked if they minded if we requested help they always answered "of course not." They just got tired of being always greeted by some of us with "Hi, Suzy, nice day isn't it...could you do me a real quick favor?" We could tell by the look on their face and other reactions when it was time "to hit up someone else next time."

The moral to these very true and common stories is to keep to a minimum the number of favors which you ask of volunteers, friends, and fellow students and workers. If the cool reaction that you receive when asking a favor seems to say that you might be wearing out your welcome, then you probably are. When this happens, find ways to predict in advance certain needs and schedule them with the PCA who gets paid for doing you favors.

And by all means, if you require a motorized mobility aid, get one. You may, at first, be concerned that you might "look more disabled" if you use a motorized wheelchair instead of a manual one. We can almost guarantee that you are the only individual around you who would feel that way; your friends and co-workers won't care what powers your 4 wheels, as long as the 4 wheels move without dependence upon these people. A primary goal of independent living is going where you wish, when you wish, and without physical dependence on others. You will appear to yourself, as well as to others around you, to be far more disabled if you are often begging pushes to destinations in your manual. The alternative is to arrive at destinations in a motorized mobility aid, on schedule and on your own, with independence from others and truly in the mainstream. Save your manual for exercise around the house and for bite-sized trips which match your strength and stamina.

Paying PCAs with Appreciation and Salary: Strategies for Expressing Appreciation

Anyone who dependably performs a service expects two types of payment...and the first type is free!

The first type of payment is given to the worker whenever the employer shows appreciation. What is appreciation? To appreciate, the dictionary tells us, "is to recognize someone's services by outwardly expressing gratitude." Gratitude speaks of "being thankful for the benefit of comforts received or discomforts relieved."

Appreciation is a very powerful force. It is so powerful an incentive that several huge agencies with very dedicated members throughout the country and the world pay no formal salaries to the majority of their workers. These are volunteer agencies which have designed and implemented highly sophisticated programs for expressing appreciation to volunteers who are willing to work long hours. These programs include certificates, pins, award banquets, media releases, and a whole hierarchy of ranked titles that the volunteers may earn by giving service.

The end objective of these costly strategies is merely to say "thank you for what you've done for me; your work is really important."

That may seem syrupy and corny, but whether workers even realize the importance of receiving appreciation, they are almost sure to lose interest in even a high-salaried job unless they regularly receive it.

The need of most workers to receive appreciation, and the employer's responsibility to provide it, are not based on the amount of salary paid to the worker. Instead, they are based upon the amount of sincere effort and high quality of work produced by the worker. Many managers mistakenly believe that by providing a worker with a decent salary, the worker is "being shown sufficient appreciation." Both minimum-wage workers as well as corporate executives require the nourishment which is supplied by routine appreciation.

Many traditional employers, who think that they must hold a reign of tight supervision and power over employees, refuse to outwardly express sincere appreciation. They usually believe that showing appreciation is to show a dependence on an employee, to therefore show weakness, and to therefore lose their sense of supervisory power and respect. Today's more modern employers, and in fact the executives of a growing number of top companies, are taking deliberate steps away from the traditional approach. These managers are outwardly expressing appreciation to employees, and the results include an increased quality of work and loyalty.

These modern managers who outwardly express appreciation find that they do not lose power and respect...on the contrary, the power and respect given to them by employees markedly increases.

As PCA managers, we should benefit from the wisdom of big business. In addition to the salaries we pay PCAs, we should outwardly express appreciation to PCAs who deserve it. As most Ph.D. psychologists will tell us, one of the most effective, powerful ways to increase the quality of services is "to positively reinforce desired behavior." If a puppy hears the evening newspaper being delivered, gets the paper, brings it to us, and we would like this to happen each evening, then the most effective way to teach the puppy is to praise him at the time we receive the newspaper.

> There are 4 main elements to powerful expressions of appreciation

When you take the time to express appreciation, you will want the expression to have a maximum positive effect on the PCA. For this to happen, you should include 4 main elements of an effective expression:

1) Express appreciation only when you sincerely mean it, and if you don't often sincerely feel appreciative of a PCA's

Methods for Paying PCAs

good-quality services, ask yourself "why not." In response, you will discover either that the PCA is doing a good job and should receive appreciation more often, or that the PCA is doing a poor job and should be corrected.

2) When you express appreciation, do it with sufficient verbal volume, speak clearly (don't mumble), and use a tone of voice which conveys the sincerity behind your expression. In the advertising business, folks have a saying which states how silly it is to have a good product to sell and not advertise it; they say "It's like blinking in the dark...if you don't tell someone, then no one will ever know what you've done." The same holds true for an expression of appreciation which the PCA doesn't hear, doesn't understand, or doesn't think is sincere...it has no positive effect.

3) When you are about to speak, lift up your chin and eyebrows, smile, and make good eye contact by looking at the PCA's eyes at a time when they are looking at yours. This visual eye and face contact with anyone to whom you want to communicate any message is a powerful way of making sure they are listening and understand your message, and it will increase the chances that they will remember your message. If you want to see this technique in action, watch any TV show where actors are speaking to each other.

4) Each effective expression of appreciation has at least 2 messages. The first message should state which service is appreciated; the second message tells the PCA why that service is important to you.

* "Earl, I am grateful for the way you clean my glasses; they really make a difference when I have to study for several hours."

The most effective expressions of appreciation have 2 main messages

* "Kathy, I like the way you hang up the towels after my shower; it's the only way they will dry out."

* "Fran, I appreciate your calling ahead tonight to tell me you would be 20 minutes late; I was able to finish some work which I must have done for a meeting tomorrow."

* "Holly, I admire the fact that you came on time tonight regardless of all the snow; that means a lot to me."

* "Dave, I want to thank you for all of the help you've given me this past year; it's wonderful to be able to depend on your help."

There is no set formula which tells us how often to show gratitude. Psychology texts do state, however, that "positive reinforcement which is randomly given is most effective." By "random," we mean "with no recognizable pattern or schedule" so that the reinforcement does not become expected on a pattern of situations or schedule.

There are four especially effective times to randomly express appreciation to PCAs:

a) Greet most arrivals of a PCA with an expression of happiness to see them or gratitude that they have arrived on time, especially if you know of a difficulty which they overcame in order to arrive such as bad weather or personal illness. "All right, there he is...wow, am I glad to see that you made it here despite all of that rain!"

b) Randomly show appreciation for work details which are done well by a current PCA who is doing a good job, by a new PCA who is learning your routine, or by a current PCA who is trying to correct bad habits. "Gee, Gordie, you learn quickly...you've been doing a great job in keeping the kitchen clean; it looks great!"

c) Show gratitude for a service which you believe has become boring, meaningless, or taken for granted by the PCA. "Gillie, I know that hanging up the bath towels to dry after my shower must seem like a small thing, but each time I need a dry towel I'm grateful that you do it."

d) Express an overall appreciation at many times when a PCA is about to leave after working a scheduled shift. "Barry, thanks a lot for your help tonight. It's very important to me. Have a great weekend and I'll look forward to seeing you on Monday night."

17. Salaries: Determining Starting Rates & Merit Increases

Routine appreciation, discussed in the previous chapter, is the first type of essential payment for PCA services, and the 2nd type of payment which each PCA expects is some form of monetary salary. In the next chapter, we will discuss both cash and noncash forms of salary. However, before we can discuss which form of salary to pay, we should determine how much of a salary to pay and how often -- if at all -- to give merit raises.

There are 2 terms which will be used in this discussion: starting rate or starting salary, and merit increase or merit raise. These are traditional terms which most people who have held jobs will quickly recognize.

Three Options for Using Starting Salaries & Merit Increases

There are at least 3 primary options for offering starting salaries and merit increases:

I
Offer the new employee an attractive starting salary and make no advance statements about any merit increases, because you don't plan to provide any increases, you are unsure whether your finances will enable you to offer future increases, or you intend to offer increases by arbitrarily deciding when to provide them as time goes on.

II
Offer the new employee an attractive starting salary and state in advance that a merit increase will be provided at specific intervals from the starting date of work.

Salaries: Determining Starting Rates & Merit Increases

III

> Offer the new employee a slightly below-average starting salary and maintain it through their orientation and training period. However, at the time of hire, announce that the first merit increase will come at the end of their orientation and training period (state a definite period of time), and that an additional merit increase will be provided at specified intervals from the starting date of work.

The first strategy is the most simple and requires the least amount of financial planning and recordkeeping. The chosen starting rate is attractive in that it matches or slightly exceeds the "going salary rate" for a similar job in your locale. Because of the 3 reasons stated in the above first strategy, you decide to make no advance promises about a possibility or schedule of future merit increases.

The second strategy is a compromise between the first and third strategies. At the time of hire, you announce that if the employee's work is satisfactory, they will receive periodic merit increases, perhaps each year on the anniversary of the starting date. For example, if an employee begins work on May 11 and their work for the following year is satisfactory, they will receive a merit increase in each future year beginning on May 11. This system requires a bit of financial planning and recordkeeping, since you want to be sure that your budget can afford to provide increases and that you will not forget to begin the promised increase on the scheduled date.

The third strategy is more complicated, however here the starting rate as well as the schedule and amount of merit increases can be coordinated to maximize financial savings to the employer. At the same time, the strategy gives the employee who is willing to stick with the job and to provide quality work an attractive merit raise package. A slight savings from this strategy can be realized by the employer:

a) By paying a minimum salary to new employees when the type of people being interviewed and hired seem to have a higher than usual potential for giving up the job or being fired within the initial period of orientation and training, and

b) By paying a minimum salary to new PCAs while they are learning the job and therefore while they are not yet working at top efficiency.

For the employer, the steps to using this third strategy include:

1) From the 3 factors outlined in the upcoming section entitled Starting Salary Rates, determine the range of starting rates which you believe you should offer.

2) Offer this starting rate, or even a slightly lower rate, for the initial orientation and trial period, and

3) When citing this starting rate to a prospective PCA, quickly add that if his work is satisfactory at the end of the initial period, he will receive his first merit increase of an amount which you specify.

For example, if most college student PCAs in your area are expecting to start at $5.00/hour, you might offer $4.75/hour during a 2-week orientation and trial period. This lower starting rate will probably be acceptable to the new PCA, because you also announce that if her work is satisfactory, she will receive her first merit increase of $.25/hour in just 2 weeks. At the end of this initial period, you add the $.25 merit increase to bring the trained and smoothly working PCA to $5.00/hour -- a salary which she will receive for an entire year, and which makes your work look more attractive over other PCA jobs.

> At least 3 factors should be considered in deciding the rate of starting salary to offer a PCA

To make this third strategy work, it is important to clearly announce the amount and date of the upcoming, first annual increase. Otherwise, the new PCA might avoid taking the job because she believes that she will be stuck for a long time with the lower, sub-average rate.

Salaries: Determining Starting Rates & Merit Increases

Starting Salary Rates

The starting rate, or starting salary, is usually an hourly rate which you have determined that you are willing and financially able to pay a newly hired PCA employee.

To determine the rate of starting salary as well as merit increases, at least three factors should be considered:

1) The salary rate which is being paid to others for doing the same or similar work in your geographical area, also known as "the going rate." Ask others who use PCAs or those who work as PCAs for advice. Don't be misled by the total rate which consumers and insurance companies are paying home health aide employment agencies, ask instead what rate the home health aide actually receives.

2) The amount of pre-existing training, skill, experience, and possible certification which is required to perform the job, i.e., is the PCA experienced and certified, or starting from scratch with no experience?

3) The amount of salary money available from the salary funding source, such as your own personal budget or a funding agency.

Since the employer will probably encounter PCA applicants who are both experienced or not experienced, a range of starting rates should be designed. For example, as of the printing date of this book, a college student with no PCA experience might expect to receive $ 5.00/hour, however a trained and certified home health aide might expect $5.50/hour. Most employers will finish their rate planning by carefully coordinating an actual starting rate with the amount and schedule of merit increases.

The overall salary goal for most employers is to pay the lowest salary possible which will result in acquiring a sufficient number of employees to provide a sufficient quality and quantity of work. To state this another way, most employers try to determine the lowest possible salary rate for which they can find enough people willing to work who will provide an acceptable quality and quantity of work.

Merit Increase Rates and Schedules

The term "merit increase" defines itself, and employees should not be allowed by an employer to confuse the term with the concept of an "automatic raise." Instead, a merit increase is an increase in salary rate which has been <u>earned</u> by the employee, and is given because the quality of work is satisfactory and merits a rate increase. It is the employer's way of telling the employee "I am pleased with your dependability, your attitude, and the quality of your work, and I am giving you a rate increase both as a reward for previous work as well as an incentive for continuing to work for me."

Increases can be given on any schedule of intervals, providing:

1) The increases are not given too frequently, so the employee loses appreciation for them just as he might if he were given a birthday party and presents each month.

2) The increases are not given too infrequently, so the employee loses interest because the increases have lost their value as a reward.

3) The amount of funding as well as the policies of any funding agency which provides you with PCA salaries, or your own financial budget, enable you to give periodic merit increases.

4) Each merit increase results in a pay rate raise which is acceptable to the source of the PCA funding and is attractive to the PCA.

5) The employer clearly states to the employee the purpose and schedule for the increases in order to maximize the benefits to the employer.

To determine the amount of merit increase to offer each time, many PCA employers and even health aide agencies follow a 3-month/anniversary/anniversary schedule. An increase of at least $.25 per hour is given at each increase date: the first increase comes after the 1st 3 months of work, and each subsequent increase comes each year on the anniversary of the worker's 1st day of employment. An increase of less than $.25 is considered to be insignificant by most employees, because this minimum means a pay raise of $10 for a 40-hour work week. Some employers also further reward their long time employees by gradually increasing the amount of each merit increase, for example offering $.25 at the first increase, $.30 at the second increase, and so forth. Some other employers have established a schedule of giving smaller merit increases each 6 months instead of a larger increase once each anniversary. Much of this innovative scheduling is based upon the amount of available budget.

18. Monetary Salaries: Cash, Noncash, or Both

To this point we have discussed whether we should use volunteers for PCA needs ("only for brief, occasional needs") and we noted that every PCA rightfully expects 2 kinds of salary: appreciation as well as a monetary salary. We outlined the why, when, and how of expressing appreciation. As an introduction to examining monetary salaries, we also studied how to set the rates for starting salaries and scheduled merit increases.

With this ground work in place, now is the time to explore monetary salaries -- their sources and the procedures, and some advantages and disadvantages of using each source.

There are 3 primary types of monetary salaries: cash, noncash, and combination of the two.

Cash Salaries

A cash salary is, in fact, seldom paid to a PCA in actual cash, but by written checks. All salaries, medical expenses, household and personal bills, and any bills sent through the mail should be paid by check. By paying salaries and bills by check, and not in green cash, you will always have proof of having made a payment. A personal checking account usually costs very little and, in fact, can actually make you money if you use an interest-bearing checking account. The use of money orders is an expensive, band-aid remedy to using personal checks. So when the term "cash salary" is used in this section, reference is made to paying PCAs by a check which they can readily convert to cash...a conversion responsibility, by the way, which is theirs and __not__ yours.

> "Cash" salaries and most routine bills should be paid by personal check and not in actual "green cash"

There are two main sources for paying a cash salary: your own personal budget and 3rd party funding.

Personal-Budget Funding for Cash Salaries

In order to have a personal budget and money in your own bank account, you might earn a regular salary from your own job, you might have compiled personal savings from whatever source, or both.

When paying for PCA salaries from your own pocket, the following procedure is common:

1) You decide the starting salary and schedule of merit increases you wish to pay,

2) Hire as many PCAs as you need and your budget allows,

3) Assign PCAs to perform any categories of duties which you require and to which they agree,

4) Keep your own time sheet and tax records for each PCA,

5) Compute, write, sign, and issue paychecks on schedule from your own bank account,

6) Compute and pay employer taxes and complete tax forms to be sent to the IRS within deadlines, and

7) Maintain your own personal budget records in order to monitor the balance of your budget and to fulfill any tax requirements.

In short, when you pay PCAs from your own personal budget, you wear the hats of a PCA manager, personnel director, foreman/supervisor, payroll clerk, bookkeeper, and tax consultant. But don't worry...you can learn all of these skills, as they apply to managing the PCAs, from this handbook!

The advantages of paying PCAs from a personal budget are several:

1) You have a clear, visible authority toward your employees, as both the source and signer of paychecks. This helps you to maintain quality control over the services you receive,

2) You can assure PCAs that paychecks will not be delayed and will be provided on schedule,

3) You have complete freedom without restrictions to hire and fire PCAs as necessary, to hire as many PCAs as you need and your budget allows, to assign any necessary categories of duties to PCAs which they agree to perform, to hire anyone you wish regardless of their training and experience, and to utilize any rate and schedule of starting salary and merit increases.

The disadvantages are few, but deserve mentioning:

1) The salaries which you pay drain your personal budget, and

2) You must keep employment records, compute salaries and payroll taxes, compute-write-sign-issue paychecks on schedule, and complete and submit employer and employee tax forms and payments according to IRS deadlines.

Let's not forget that if you are mentally able and willing to perform these and other management duties, but you lack the physical abilities or stamina to do so, then there is no reason to surrender your management control and move from the driver's seat to a backseat passenger slot. As we discussed in the chapter "The 3 Management Situations: Which Applies to Me?," it might be appropriate to hire a PCA Coordinator to physically carry out those particular management chores which you are unable to perform. Just like a Lee Iacocca or any other executive, you are still clearly the manager-in-charge, however you have hired a coordinator to carry out your instructions in certain areas. More details on the role and hiring of a PCA Coordinator are found in the chapter of this book on "The 3 Management Situations... ".

3rd-Party Funding For Cash Salaries

The second possible source for paying a cash salary is by receiving 3rd party funding. The term "3rd party funding" is quite common. Here it refers to the situation where you are the 1st party, the PCA (the recipient of the money) is the 2nd, and the funding source is the 3rd party. The term is also

Monetary Salaries: Cash, Noncash, or Both 201

commonly used by dealers of medical goods when they ask "Will you be paying cash for this (wheelchair), or will we be billing a 3rd party source." For PCA salaries, the 3rd party funding usually comes from health or disability insurance, or a federal governmental agency such as Medicaid, Medicare, Social Security, Veterans Affairs, a state Office for Vocational Rehabilitation (OVR or DVR), or a county or city health department.

If you wish to pay for PCA salaries from 3rd party funding, the following procedure shows some typical steps to becoming eligible with a funding source. Just as there are many possible funding sources, there are just as many possible procedures in becoming established and eligible with a source. The following 5-step procedure is merely an example:

1) You inquire about your eligibility for any funding which can be used to pay PCA salaries. Inquiries are made with the insurance agents where you have health insurance policies and at various county, state, and federal agencies,

2) When a potential source is found, you apply for the funding and become eligible for benefits,

3) You learn about the restrictions and step-by-step procedures for hiring and paying PCAs whom you use,

4) You (or a home health aide agency required by the funding source) hire and pay PCAs according to the prescribed restrictions and procedures, and

5) You respond periodically to the funding source's review of your continued financial eligibility for their program.

> There are at least 4 common routes which 3rd parties use for paying PCAs: you should know the advantages & disadvantages of the route assigned to you

Once you are eligible to receive funding, several possible ways exist for receiving it. Four of the most frequently used routes are outlined below. The actual restrictions and step-by-step route to be used by a source is purely their decision...after all, if they are giving you money then they should have the right to stipulate how you will receive and spend it. Also, keep in mind that we have loosely referred to you "receiving funding"; in actuality, you might receive paid services but never see the actual money because most funding sources will pay the PCAs directly.

Here are 4 common routes chosen by funding sources for paying PCAs:

1) In this first example, the 3rd party gives actual money to you, you deposit it into your bank account, you hire and pay PCAs with checks from this account, and you supply the funding source with items of documentation which they request, such as signed forms or copies of cancelled checks, that prove that payments were made.

From your perspective, this is the most desirable route although it is infrequently used by funding sources since it is most open to abuse of the funds. When used, this route gives you most of the same freedoms, authority, and advantages as paying PCAs from your personal budget.

2) In a second example, you are instructed by the funding source to hire PCAs and to sign and submit timesheets which request the processing of paychecks. The funding source will then either send you agency-signed checks to hand to PCAs or they will send checks directly to PCAs.

This is a common method used by funding sources. It gives you many of the same advantages as paying by personal funds, except that the paychecks are sometimes delayed in arriving from the funding source. The source will also usually dictate the salary rate as well as whether and when merit increases can be given.

If you are given a choice of receiving checks which you hand to PCAs or having them send checks directly to PCAs, choose the first method for 2 advantages. You will know right away whether the paychecks the PCA expects are arriving on schedule, and the mechanical process of your handing each check to the PCA gives you an added image of authority for controlling the schedule and quality of services you receive.

3) With a third possible route for payments, you are instructed to hire PCAs and to submit to the funding source the names of the PCAs as well as standard number of hours which will apply to every pay period that each PCA is expected to work. The source then sends a paycheck each time for payment of this number of "contract hours" to you or to each PCA.

Because it lacks flexibility, this method is less desirable and is becoming less frequently used by funding sources. PCAs seldom work a "contract, standard number of work hours" due to the unpredictable nature of the exact duration of help you require from day to day. Consequently, this method often results in under and over payments of PCAs and results either in PCA complaints, when underpaid, or in a decreasing amount of authority for you when the PCA realizes that she will be paid the contract amount regardless of whether or not she works the full number of hours or her work is satisfactory.

4) A fourth funding route is characterized by a set of severe restrictions. The 3rd party requires you to use a home health aide agency which takes over most of the management and payment functions. The agency often first evaluates your medical records and on-site needs and then issues its opinion about which categories of assistance you will receive, the number of hours of assistance you require, and the schedule for which that help will be supplied. The agency then hires, pays, and schedules PCAs to provide you with assistance.

This method is frequently used by governmental funding agencies and is the least desirable method for those who are able and willing to independently manage and otherwise have quality control over the PCAs they hire. However, for those who are unable or unwilling to manage PCAs, the required use of home health aide agencies is essential.

With any of these four methods, the most obvious advantage of using a 3rd party funding source is that funding comes from the source and not from your personal budget. In addition, you seldom have any IRS paperwork or employer/employee taxes to pay because the agency assumes that responsibility.

The disadvantages of 3rd party regulation of PCA funding depend upon whether you are mentally and emotionally able and willing to be in control and manage the PCAs you use. If you find that you or a family member cannot realistically manage your PCAs, for whatever reason, then the 4th option -- that of 3rd party management -- will probably be the most appealing. In contrast, if you are able and willing to manage help to the maximum extent possible, then the restrictions which often come with 3rd party funding may be annoying or even completely intolerable to you.

Depending on the route of funding and the policies of any home health aide agency used, these restrictions can include your lack of freedom to hire and fire as needed, to hire the number of PCAs you needed, to assign certain necessary categories of duties, to set salary or merit increase rates and schedules, or to have the authority necessary for asserting quality control for the assistance you receive.

> Often a noncash salary will not cost you anything, because you are sharing something valuable which you already own or must otherwise purchase for yourself

Additional disadvantages of 3rd party management of funding might include the periodic paperwork required by the funding source regarding your continued financial and medical eligibility for their program, as well as their evaluations of your continued types and durations of need for PCA assistance. As mentioned, there may also be occasional or frequent delays in paychecks when they come from a funding source. If you use 3rd party funding, and paychecks will be issued for PCAs whom you hire, inquire about the usual paycheck delivery schedule that the source intends to follow. Be sure to discuss this intended schedule with the PCAs, and then tell them not to be disappointed when delays that occur are beyond your control.

Noncash Salaries

A noncash salary is payment in a form other than money (or check). It can be some service or material benefit that is equal to or is of even greater value than the amount which would otherwise be paid in cash. These services or benefits usually center around sharing your living space with a live-in PCA. However, your innovative thinking about your abilities to provide attractive services, or about your desire to share some of your possessions. can often create noncash salaries which do not require sharing living space.

Many people who must pay for assistance from their pockets have found that they could not possibly pay for all of their PCA needs without using noncash salaries.

There are 3 main circumstances when you might wish to consider paying a noncash salary. Each circumstance addresses a time when 3rd party funding is either not available or not desirable, and one would therefore be forced otherwise to use cash from one's personal budget. In short, if you are receiving 3rd party funding for all of your PCA needs and you are satisfied with the payment system and its restrictions, then you probably have little need to consider a noncash salary. We suggest, however, that you be familiar with its potential for possible needs in the future.

The use of noncash salaries should be considered when:

1) 3rd party funding is not available,

2) 3rd party funding is not desirable because of its restrictions,

3) 3rd party funding is available for only part of your needs and a personal budget must be used for the other categories of needs, or

4) Your personal budget cannot be stretched to cover all your PCA needs.

The procedure for establishing a noncash salary system is rather simple:

1) Compute the value of the desired starting salary and the schedule and amounts of any merit increases as if you were intending to pay cash salaries,

2) List the possible noncash services or benefits which you could offer a PCA,

3) Next to each possible service or benefit, list its monetary value,

4) Choose the service(s) or benefit(s) that are equal or slightly greater in value to the starting salary you computed in step one, above, and

5) For the first merit increase, list an additional service or benefit which is equal or greater to the monetary value of the first merit increase you computed in step one, above.

In deciding which services or benefits to offer as noncash salary items, we suggest that the following 8 considerations should be made:

1) Consider items which are attractive to the PCA because they fulfill a living need which they have,

> Consider the probable age and lifestyle of the type of PCA you will be hiring and determine which items or services might be attractive for their personal needs. If you have extra living space in your apartment, condo, or house, you might consider offering a rent-free live-in offer as partial or total payment to a PCA for services. For quarters you are renting, determine the fair-market value of the live-in quarters by consulting your apartment rent lease. On the other hand, if you own the condo or house or are paying a mortgage on it, ask a local realtor about the fair-market rent value for the size and type of living space which you are offering. See the 2 chapters "Tax Obligations for a PCA Employer" and "Medical Deductions & Credits" for details about deducting the value of live-in quarters as a medical expense on your federal income taxes.
>
> Be careful to choose a personally compatible and honest individual for your live-in help. State in writing on the job description any agreements regarding specific hours

Monetary Salaries: Cash, Noncash, or Both

(if any) in which the PCA can share your own living space, rules about parties and whether the PCA is allowed to offer either an overnight or long-term sharing of his space to his friends, the use or borrowing of your possessions, whether smoking, drugs, or alcohol is allowed, understandings about food preparation and storage areas, and use of the telephone. Also in the written job description, be sure to stipulate that a live-in PCA who is fired or resigns must vacate immediately on ending their assistance to you.

2) Consider only those noncash benefits that are acceptable to you because they do not significantly jeopardize your privacy or security of possessions,

>Poor choices might include sharing all parts of your house on a 24-hour basis. Instead, clearly define the speceific house entrance, bedroom, and bathroom that the PCA may use as well as the hours to which kitchen privileges apply.

3) Consider items which have a clear, definite value,

>Good choices include sharing an apartment for which you pay a specific rent, or allowing the PCA to occupy a room in your house after checking with area realtors regarding the local fair renting value for such a room.

> Choose noncash items of a fixed, definite value which cannot be inflated or damaged by a PCA's extensive or inconsiderate use

4) Consider items with a definite value which cannot be abused or inflated by the PCA,

>Poor choices would include agreeing to pay for all of the PCA's food or telephone toll calls. If offering these items is attractive to you, place a clear maximum on the value of your liability, for example, "the 1st $20 per week of food," or "the 1st $20 per month of toll calls which you make." In the future, these maximum values can be gradually increased in stages as the noncash equivalent to monetary merit increases.

5) Consider providing items with a definite value which can be documented by printed receipts if their value is to be declared as medical deductions on personal income taxes (for details on taking such deductions, see the 2 sections on Taxes).

> Good choices for noncash salaries include rent which is stipulated in a lease and for which you pay by check each month, or utilities for which a bill is received and for which you pay by check. For items for which you receive a routine bill, compute the average monthly cost for the item and then divide the monthly cost by the number of people who have equal use of the item. For example, if rent for your 2 bedroom apartment costs $600 per month and you plan to share it with 2 PCAs, then each of the 3 of you would ordinarily pay $200 per month as roommates. Offering a PCA free rent in exchange for doing PCA work is therefore a noncash equivalent to $200 in hourly wages per month. If you would be paying a cash hourly wage of $4 per hour, then the $200 rent benefit is payment for 50 hours of work each month, or 12.5 hours per week.

> Be sure to check with tax authorities before implementing any plan which involves declaring PCA expenses as medical deductions. They, and not this book, have the authority to approve of your plan.

You can similarly add up and average the monthly cost for such items as utilities (heat, electricity, and water and sewer), property taxes, and telephone. For telephone bills, consider offering to pay a share of the fixed monthly service charge, and not the variable amount for toll calls.

For example, perhaps the standard monthly service charge (including all taxes) for the shared telephone is $24.00. If you and 2 live-in PCAs share this phone, and you agree to pay this standard charge, then each PCA is receiving a noncash salary of $8.00 per month. We advise that when each month's phone bill arrives, each PCA pays you for each toll call which she has made.

6) Consider items which cannot be easily physically abused or damaged by PCAs,

It is not wise to give a PCA open use of such items as your stereo or record-tape-CD collection, or use of your car when you are not a passenger.

7) Prioritize those items which you either already own or on which you are already making payments, and which you can share at little or no additional cost to you,

If you rent a 2-bedroom apartment or own a 3 bedroom house, and a bedroom is not used, consider offering a live-in position to a PCA.

8) Besides considering physical items, create a list of services which you can perform and offer to a PCA as noncash payment.

These services can easily be assigned a fair-market pricetag and might include professional services such as typing, phone answering, bookkeeping, computer work, or tax preparation for which you are trained; babysitting; academic tutoring or skills which a PCA wants and you can teach; transportation which you can provide; shopping or errands which you can perform; or household services such as sewing or homecooked meals which you can provide for an appreciative PCA.

19. U.S. Tax Obligations for a PCA Employer

In the U.S., it is important to understand and meet your tax obligations when you directly employ PCAs and pay their salaries directly from your personal budget. These tax obligations address completing and filing reports about your employment of PCAs as well as computing and paying actual taxes. As an employer, you might have only employer-related obligations in some circumstances, while in others you might be responsible for both employer and employee-related obligations. These circumstances and obligations will be explained.

> Before we start, please note that the following sections provide merely an introduction to tax information about employing PCAs for personal needs. The information is intended as only a guideline and not as legal advice. As a brief introduction, this information might be incomplete or out of date for your complex personal needs, regardless of the extensive research which went into compiling this data. Before proceeding to file or pay any employer taxes (or deciding not to so so), you should obtain updated and complete details from IRS publications, IRS technical assistance staff, and perhaps an accountant or tax preparer whom you consult.

In general, you directly employ PCAs when they are hired, supervised, and paid by you and not by an agency or someone else. If an agency employs and supplies the PCAs you use, then you are probably not a direct employer and have no tax obligations. However, if the agency merely gives you a list of PCAs and you then contact, hire, and pay PCAs from that list, then those individuals are probably your direct employees. In either case, you should confirm the facts by simply asking the agency or IRS technical assistance whether you have any tax obligations to Uncle Sam.

You are considered to be paying PCA salaries from your personal budget when the money comes from the earnings or savings in your personal bank account, and you are not reimbursed for all or part of those salaries by an outside, 3rd-party funding source. If you are reimbursed, or if a

Tax Obligations for a PCA Employer

funding source directly pays each PCA with paychecks which it signs and issues, then ask that funding source whether you have any tax obligations.

If, however, you do directly employ and pay the PCAs who assist you, then you have a good chance of having tax obligations. We advise that you read the following sections and then either legally avoid tax obligations by structuring your method of employing PCAs, or that you legally meet your obligations by filing reports and making tax payments.

First, if you pay PCA salaries out of your personal budget, you may be tempted to simply pay PCAs by handing them greenback cash and therefore forgetting about all hassels of filing reports, paying taxes, and keeping records. "Paying under the table" seems so simple and easy for both you and the PCAs.

There are two concerns with paying salaries with this "under the table" approach First, if the IRS catches you with their increasing computer capabilities, there may be considerable penalties involved for charges of tax evasion or fraud. These penalties can be applied to you, the employer, for not reporting wages which you pay, and to the PCAs, your employees, for not reporting the wages they earn.

Second, whether you are paying from your pocket a large or small sum of wages each year for PCA assistance, you should take advantage of medically-related deductions for these salaries on your personal income tax. Just as medical deductions include health insurance premiums, prescription medications, and some physician prescribed medical equipment and supplies, the salaries you pay PCAs -- cash and noncash -- usually qualify as medically-related deductions from income taxes. It's a shame to pay more personal income tax than the amount for which you are legally required.

Most of us who earn our own living without payments from 3rd party funding programs must pay personal income taxes. We work hard to make our personal budget cover our living costs, and we want to legally avoid paying as much income tax as possible. Therefore, it is advisable to spend the time to learn about tax obligations and taking medical deductions in order to avoid overpaying taxes.

The catch to being able to deduct PCA salaries as medical expenses is that the salaries can't be paid under-the-table. Uncle Sam insists that if someone wishes to benefit from deducting salaries as medical expenses, they must first file forms to report paying the salaries and then must pay certain employer taxes on those salaries. Details about ways to claim PCA medical expenses as tax deductions are found in the next chapter of this book, "Medical Deductions & Credits for PCA Employers."

> By understanding your tax obligations, you might be able to legally avoid some tax requirements by carefully structuring the way in which you personally employ PCAs

The primary cost, then, of jumping through all the IRS hoops is in terms of time:

a) Taking the time to understand which IRS forms and employer tax requirements apply to you,

b) Setting up a basic recordkeeping system and maintaining a supply of applicable IRS forms, and

c) Taking the time to complete the required forms, compute and pay the employer taxes, and submit the forms and payments within the IRS-stated deadlines.

Here's how it is done.

Kinds of Employees Whom You Directly Employ

There are 3 primary categories of employees whom you are most likely to employ for PCA help: independent contractors, household employees, and family members.

Independent Contractors. Some PCAs who are business-minded might make their services available to you and to others on a contracted basis. Like lawyers, carpenters, and many household maids, these PCAs contract their services.

Tax Obligations for a PCA Employer

These people have received previous training in their profession, and you offer them work and brief them on the type of work you want done. You both agree on a standard work schedule for each day and a standard weekly or monthly amount or fee they will be paid if their work is satisfactory. Contracted workers are usually paid a contracted fee for services instead of an hour-by-hour rate, eventhough that fee is usually initially computed by considering the hours of work required for the fee. Periodically, the independent contractor will give you a bill and you pay the flat fee requested in return for the dates of service stated on the bill.

In Publication 539, the IRS cites a guideline regarding their definition of an independent contractor:

> The general rule of thumb is that an individual is an independent contractor if you, the employer, have the right to control or direct only the result of the work and not the means and methods of accomplishing the result.

Whether this guideline applies to the way in which you employ PCAs is a decision you must make. As we shall see in a minute, independent contractors -- and not the employers who receive their bills and pay their fees -- are responsible for their own tax obligations. However, if you pay any non-corporate contractor $600 or more within any year you must file an IRS Form 1099-MISC, which merely states the total fees you paid him.

Household Employees. The second type of employee with which we are concerned is termed by the IRS a "household employee." The IRS defines these as "persons you hire to perform services in and about your private home." If you consider your home to be your current place of residence, then PCAs whom you directly employ while temporarily living in a college dormitory or apartment could probably also be considered household employees. In any case, these are folks you actually employ; "household employee" requirements do not usually apply to independent contractors who perform work in your home.

In Publication 503, the IRS states the following as an introduction to your tax obligations toward this category of worker. Their use of the term "may" refers to your having different obligations toward them in different circumstances. If you employ only a couple of part-time PCAs, you might not need to pay certain taxes which are required when employing several part-time or any number of full-time PCAs. This advantageous (and legal) structuring of your PCA employment will be described later in this section.

If you have a household employee, you may be subject to Social Security Tax (FICA). You may also have to pay Federal Unemployment Tax (FUTA). This is for your employee's unemployment insurance. If your employee asks you to withhold income tax and you agree, you will be subject to income tax withholding.

As mentioned, some employment taxes can be legally avoided by hiring part-time PCAs. Employers are required to pay most types of employment taxes (especially FICA and FUTA taxes) when the wages paid to a worker exceed specified amounts during a specified number of months.

For example, an employer must pay FICA (federal Social Security) taxes whenever a worker's wages exceed $50 in any 3-month calendar quarter. (The 4 IRS calendar quarters are Jan-Feb-Mar, Apr-May-Jun, Jul-Aug-Sep, and Oct-Nov-Dec). If an employer limits some or all workers to part-time hours, and each worker earns less than $50 in wages during a calendar quarter, then the employer legally avoids paying FICA taxes for those workers during that quarter.

FUTA (federal unemployment) taxes can be legally avoided in any calendar quarter when household-employee PCAs, collectively, are paid less than $1,000 in cash wages during that calendar quarter.

For both FICA and FUTA taxes, only cash wages are counted; non-cash wages are not. Other advantages of dividing your needs among several part-time PCAs are discussed in the chapter "Dividing Needs with More Than One PCA." Paying noncash wages are further explained in "Monetary Salaries: Cash, Noncash, or Both."

Family Members. This 3rd category of help comes from family members. It is possible to receive services from a child, who works for her parent, or from a spouse. If these people are paid a salary, the IRS states the following in Publication 539 as an introduction to employer tax obligations:

> The services of a child under the age of 21 who works for his or her parent and the services of an individual who works for his or her spouse are not covered (usually) by social security or federal unemployment. This is true even if the child or the individual is paid regular wages. Their wages are not subject to social security and federal unemployment taxes. But their wages may still be subject to income tax withholding.

For any of these 3 types of workers, the IRS states, in Publication 539,

> there is no difference between full-time and part-time employees. You must figure the social security and federal unemployment taxes (when required) for part-time workers or workers hired for short periods the same way as for full-time workers. It does not matter whether the worker has another job or is having the maximum amount of social security tax withheld by another employer. Income tax withholding may be figured the same way as for full-time workers, or it may be figured by the part-year employment method.

Knowing your obligations, when paying cash or noncash wages

Your tax obligations will be different depending upon whether you pay cash or noncash wages.

Definitions and examples of cash and non-cash wages are discussed in the chapter "Monetary Salaries: Cash, Noncash, or Both." The following sections are separated according to these 2 areas.

Knowing your obligations -- when paying cash wages

■ Identification Numbers. Both an employer and each employee should have separate, personal, lifetime identification numbers issued by the government. For the employer, the number is called an Employer Identification Number (EIN) and is acquired by completing a Form SS-4. For the employee, the number is called a Social Security Number and is acquired by filing a Form SS-5.

■ Social Security (FICA). Employers who pay cash salaries of $50 or more in any IRS defined calendar quarter are required to file Form 942 and to pay FICA (Federal Insurance Contributions Act) tax. The IRS defines the calendar quarters to be Jan-Feb-Mar, Apr-May-Jun, Jul-Aug-Sep, and Oct-Nov-Dec. As an example, the rate in 1988 is 15.02% of cash wages. One-half, or 7.51%, is withheld from the employee's paycheck; the employer usually contributes the other half. Employers should check with a nearby Social Security office to determine the current rate and requirements in effect. FICA taxes, due within 30 days after the end of each quarter, are sent along with a completed Form 942. Employers of independent contractors or family members are usually not responsible for these taxes.

> For further details on types of tax obligations, forms, filing deadlines, and procedures, consult IRS publications (free), IRS technical assistance (free), or a tax preparer whom you employ

■ Federal Income Tax. Employers of household help may choose to either withhold or not withhold federal income tax from employee paychecks. The IRS tells us that an employee must request these withholdings and an employer must agree to withhold before the obligation exists. Few employers of household help decide to withhold tax. Employers of independent contractors or family members are usually not responsible for these taxes.

■ Form W-2. Regardless of whether federal income tax is withheld, employers must file an annual W-2 form for each household employee. The form must include the value of all wages paid, cash or noncash. It will also require the value of all cash wages which were subject to FICA (Social Security) taxes. Employers of independent contractors or family members are usually not responsible for this reporting.

Tax Obligations for a PCA Employer

■ Form 1099-MISC. The employer of an independent contractor, who pays a non-corporate contractor $600 or more in any year, must file this annual form which states the total of wages paid.

■ Federal and State Unemployment Taxes. If you paid cash wages of $1,000 or more to household employees in any calendar quarter of the current or preceding year, you are liable for FUTA (Federal Unemployment Tax Act) tax on any employees you have in the current year. Unlike Social Security tax which is usually shared between employer and employee, the entire FUTA tax is the financial responsibility of the employer. Payments are reported to the IRS on Form 940. Employers should check with the IRS to determine the current FUTA rate and requirements in effect.

In addition to this Federal tax, most states also require a separate unemployment tax. To satisfy state obligations, new employers are usually charged a fairly high initial rate. Their subsequent rate is determined by the employer's track record with workers -- if the employer fires many workers and they are successful at filing for unemployment benefits, the employer's rate rises; if not, the rate decreases. Employers should consult their state's department of labor for current rates and requirements.

■ Workers' Compensation and Disability Benefits Insurances.

Workers' compensation insurance pays an employee medical benefits and a portion of their salary for the duration of an illness or injury which is caused by their job or which occurs on their job site. Disability benefits insurance pays a portion of salary to an employee during an illness or injury which is not job related.

Both of these closely related insurances are often required by state laws, and the employer purchases the insurance by paying periodic premiums to a commercial carrier of their choice. The requirements, which are stipulated by state law, vary from state to state and can be obtained by calling any state's department of labor.

In some states, a home health aide agency is required to supply the insurances for employees, however the private individual who will be personally employing aides in his home as domestic help is not required to provide these particular insurances when "domestic ('around the house') employees are employed less than 40 hours per week." Check your own state's requirements.

Many private individuals who insure their rented or purchased living quarters will find that limited workers' compensation coverage is included in their renter's or homeowner's insurance coverage. An increasing number of policies are including workman's compensation insurance for part time employees who are employed at a residence for non-commercial, not-for-profit purposes. So if your policy includes this coverage, and a PCA injures himself while physically helping you or mowing your lawn, you might be covered for the medical expenses incurred by your employee. Check your policy.

Knowing your obligations -- when paying noncash wages

■ Identification Numbers. [see the previous section for cash wages]

■ Form W-2. [see the previous section for cash wages]

■ Form 1099-MISC. Those who pay noncash wages such as rents, utilities, services, and similar items to household employees are required to file this annual form which states the fair-market, cash value of the noncash wages that were paid.

■ Workers' Compensation and Disability Benefits Insurances. [see the previous section for cash wages]

Record Keeping Strategies

For Cash & Noncash Wages. Keep for at least 4 years all records of employment taxes which you pay. These should be available for IRS review if requested. We suggest that you keep printed records which document and prove the following categories of information:

Tax Obligations for a PCA Employer 219

■ Your employer identification number
■ Amounts and dates of all wage payments
■ Receipts and statements which prove the fair-market value of all noncash wages paid: rent receipts, utility bills, telephone bills, food receipts, and other statements
■ Cancelled checks and money-order receipts which prove that cash salaries were paid, employment taxes were paid, and bills were paid to supply noncash salary benefits
■ Names, addresses, and social security numbers of employees
■ Beginning and ending dates of employment for each employee
■ Dates and amounts of employment taxes which you paid
■ The "payer's copy," if provided, or photo copy of each tax document which you complete and send to the Social Security Administration or IRS

If you will be subject to meeting deadlines for tax payments and filing documents, we suggest keeping a tax calendar. This is simply marking any commonly used reference calendar or appointment book one year in advance with at least the following details:

a) The dates on which various forms will be due at various government offices,
b) Consequently, the dates by which forms should be put in the mail in order to reach those offices by their deadline dates,
c) Which forms are due on each of these dates, and
d) To which agency the forms and payments should be sent.

Noncash Wage Record Card. When noncash wages are paid to a PCA, such as supplying rent, utilities, telephone, or food, we suggest that the employer has each PCA sign a noncash wage record card each year or at the termination of their employment (whichever occurs first).

This card provides a clear record of the specific noncash wage items and their cash value which were received by each PCA. Since this value is usually a medically-deductible expense on the employer's personal income tax, this card is a very valuable summary statement. It can be shown to the IRS as proof of the value of the noncash wage, as well as the "nursing-like" type of work performed, in the event that the employer's tax records are audited. For an explanation of the importance of using the term "nursing-like duties," please see the chapter of this book, "Medical Deductions & Credits for PCA Employers."

An ordinary index card may be used with information such as the following typed onto it. The informal wording below which appears in parentheses ( ) should not appear on the finished card. Instead, the types of information stated here in the parentheses should be substituted to apply to your particular situation. You should feel free to change this information as it applies to the specific noncash salary which you have offered. The PCA should sign the card as certification that the noncash wage was received and that other information is correct. One card per PCA should be completed by the employer and signed by each PCA, either at the end of each calendar year or at the end of a PCA's employment, whichever occurs first.

Index Card Outline

> (the date of the end of employment or December 31)
>
> This is to certify that I, (PCA's full name), performed medical attendant services for (your full name), (brief statement of medical condition, such as "a quadriplegic who uses a wheelchair"). For these nursing-like duties, not to include household chores, I received the benefits of a noncash salary consisting of (state the noncash items "paid" to the PCA and the value of each, such as "my share of the rent (state the monthly amount) and utilities from (state the beginning and ending dates of employment). (Your name) paid these bills on my behalf, and the total value of the noncash wages was ($ total).
>
> (PCA's typed name, home address, social security #)
>
> (PCA's signature)

Completed Card Example

> 11/30/86
>
> This is to certify that I, Scott Downs, performed medical attendant services for Earl Krystal, a quadriplegic who uses a wheelchair. For these nursing-like duties, not to include household chores, I received the benefits of a noncash salary consisting of my share of the rent ($630 monthly / 3 roommates) and utilities ($1170 for 10 months / 3 roommates) from 2/1/86 to 11/30/86.
> Mr. Krystal paid these bills on my behalf, and the total value of the noncash wages was $2100 rent + $390 utilities = $2490.
>
> Scott Downs
> 91 Bay State Road   (Scott Downs' signature)
> Carbondale, IL 62901
> 074-69-2523

20. Medical Deductions & Credits for PCA Employers (U.S.)

This section provides a brief introduction to information about claiming PCA employment expenses as medically related deductions from income taxes in the U.S.

Before reading this chapter, please keep in mind:

a) The information in this section is taken from Internal Revenue Service (IRS) publications. These publications are available to anyone at no charge. For a listing of the titles and numbers of those IRS publications of special interest to those who incur disability and health-related expenses, as well as details on how to obtain this literature, please refer to the chapter of this book entitled "A Listing of U.S. Tax Publications for PCA Employers."

b) The information in this chapter is purposely brief and intended to introduce you to topics of special concern to you. This brevity is due to the frequent changes that occur in U.S. tax laws. We believe that it is better to introduce the reader here to certain topics and then refer to sources where up-to-date details can be readily found, instead of printing details in this book which might soon be outdated by new tax laws or interpretations.

c) Consequently, the information in this section should be considered merely as a guideline, and not as legal advice or interpretation of tax law. We advise anyone who has concerns about complex medical deductions and related recordkeeping to consult a reputable tax preparer and to obtain IRS technical assistance.

According to the IRS, "Medical expenses are payments you make for the diagnosis, treatment, or prevention of disease. They also include payments you make for treatment affecting any part or function of the body. Include in medical expenses the cost of transportation for needed medical care. Also include payments for medical insurance that provides coverage for yourself, your spouse, and dependents. There are limits on amounts you may deduct."

The IRS publication "Tax Information for Handicapped and Disabled Individuals" further provides lists of medical expenses which do qualify for medical deductions and those which do not qualify.

Deducting PCA Cash & Noncash Salaries

One of the medical expenses which is usually deductible, that of medical care, is covered in this publication by a section which addresses attendant wages:

> Wages (are deductible) for an attendant who provides nursing services. You also may include in medical expenses other amounts you paid for nursing services, including amounts you paid for the attendant's meals. Services need not be performed by a nurse as long as the services are of a kind generally performed by a nurse. This includes services connected with caring for the patient's condition, such as giving medication or changing dressings, as well as the bathing and grooming of the patient.
>
> Divide the food expense among the household members to find the cost of the attendant's food. If you had to pay additional amounts for household upkeep because of the attendant, include as a medical expense the extra amount you paid. This includes items such as extra rent you paid because you moved to a larger apartment to provide space for the attendant, or the extra cost of utilities for the attendant. If the attendant also provided personal and household services, you must further divide these amounts between the time spent in performing household and other personal services and the time spent on nursing services. Only the amount spent for nursing services is a medical care expense.
>
> [In addition to tax deductions] certain expenses for household services or for the care of a qualifying individual incurred to enable the taxpayer to be gainfully employed may qualify for the child and dependent care credit, explained later in this [IRS] publication.

Tax Credits for PCA Services

The tax credit to which reference is made above may be taken if you pay someone for nursing services which then enables you (or your spouse if you are married) to work or look for work.

If you pay someone to care for your dependent who is under 15, your disabled dependent, or your disabled spouse so that you can work or look for work, then you may be able to take a tax credit of up to 30% of the amount you pay. You may use up to $2,400 of these expenses to figure your credit if you have one qualifying dependent and up to $4,800 if you have two or more qualifying dependents. Your credit can consequently range from $720 to as much as $1440.

If you pay someone to look after your dependent or spouse in your home, you may be a household employer. See [the IRS Publication #503] "Employment Taxes for Household Employers" for a discussion on how to figure employment taxes and what forms you must file if you are a household employer.

This IRS Publication 503 provides considerable more detail regarding definitions and other conditions which qualify for this advantageous tax credit.

PCA Services as Medical or Business-Related Deductions

Another topic that this particular publication addresses is which expenses are medically deductible when traveling with a friend or spouse who performs PCA services. At some times these services are considered medical expenses, and at others they are categorized as business expenses. Again, to quote from publication 503:

> Example 1. You are blind and to do your work you must use a reader. You use the reader both during your regular working hours at your place of work and outside of your regular working hours away from your place of work. The reader's services are only for your work. You may deduct your expenses for the reader as employee business expenses.

Medical Deductions & Credits for PCA Employers

Example 2. You are confined to a wheelchair. Sometimes you must go out of town on business. Your friend or spouse goes with you to help with such things as carrying your luggage or getting up steps. You do not pay your helper a salary, but you do pay for your helper's travel, meals, and lodging while on such trips. In your home town you do your job without a helper. Because the expenses for travel, meals, and lodging of your helper are directly related to doing your job, you may deduct them as employee business expenses.

Example 3. You are confined to a wheelchair. You must go on overnight out-of-town business trips as a part of your job. Your friend goes with you on these trips to help with your wheelchair, your luggage, and your daily medications. You do not pay a salary to your friend. You do pay for all your friend's travel, meals, and lodging while on these trips. However, you also need your friend's help regularly during the hours you are not working, while at home and out-of-town. The expenses for the travel, meals, and lodging of your friend are nursing services. You include them as medical expenses.

If, instead of your friend, your spouse goes with you on the out of town business trips, you may deduct as medical expenses only the out-of-pocket expenses for your spouse's travel. Expenses for your spouse's meals and lodging are not deductible.

In summary, this section has introduced you to some of the tax deductions and credits which apply to the medical expenses of your paying for PCA help. Remember that any expenses not paid by you, because the paychecks come from someone else or an agency, are not deductible by you. This also applies to medical expenses which you initially pay and for which you are reimbursed at a later date.

Of course, there are many additional categories of deductible medical expenses, such as prescription medications, medical equipment, and health insurance premiums. We have addressed only those related to hiring PCA help. The free IRS publications in the listing found in the next chapter provide considerable detail for all areas.

21. A Listing of U.S. Tax Publications for PCA Employers

The following publications are available free for the asking at most offices of the U.S. Internal Revenue Service. Before making a trip to an office, check your phone book's blue pages section on "U.S. Government." There may be toll free numbers for the Internal Revenue Service or the Social Security Administration. Among these numbers many cities list a separate number for mail-ordering forms and publications.

With the previous chapter's explanation of several forms and the following bibliography of free publications, you will know exactly what to request.

■ "Employer's Tax Guide - Circular E," Publication 15

■ "Medical and Dental Expenses," publication 502

■ "Child and Dependent Care Credit, and Employment Taxes for Household Employers," Publication 503

■ "Credit for the Elderly or for the Permanently and Totally Disabled," Publication 524

■ "Taxable and Nontaxable Income," Publication 525

■ "Recordkeeping for Individuals and a List of Tax Publications," Publication 552

■ "Employment Taxes: Employees Defined, Income Tax Withholding, Social Security Taxes (FICA), Federal Unemployment Tax (FUTA), and Reporting and Allocating Tips," Publication 539

■ "Tax Information for Handicapped and Disabled Individuals," Publication 907

■ "Taxpayer's Guide to IRS Information, Assistance, and Publications," Publication 910

Section V

Recruiting, Interviewing, Training, & Parting with Help

22) Creating a Job Description for PCAs

23) Residence Locations for a PCA

24) Sources for Recruiting PCAs

25) Methods for Recruiting PCAs

26) Interviewing, Screening, & Hiring Prospective PCAs

27) Training & Ongoing Management

28) Predicting, Recognizing, and Resolving PCA Problems

29) Parting Ways from a PCA

30) 10 Top Guidelines for Maximum Independent Living

22. Creating a Job Description for PCAs

The Importance of a Job Description

Before the construction developer of a new shopping mall can start to order actual building materials, she must develop a planning document on paper. This planning tool includes the name of the new shopping center; a description of its size, shape, and marketing image; detailed blueprints of the stores to be built; and a few summary remarks. No construction developer would think of ordering concrete and building blocks before this planning document was in writing.

Before a PCA employer or manager can start recruiting, interviewing, hiring, or training employees, he must develop a similar planning document about the title for the employees to be hired, a description of the nature of the work to be performed, the detailed "blueprint" list of specific duties to be performed, and a few summary remarks which clarify work hours and salary. No PCA employer or manager should think of starting to recruit PCA employees before this planning document is in writing.

> Don't try to remember all the details of a job description in your head unless your routine is very brief-- a well written description, like a building contractor's blueprint, makes managing easier for you because the duties are clear to you & to the PCA

For the employer and manager, this document is called a job description. Just as a construction developer, architect, or contractor would not consider trying to keep all the building details in his head, a written planning document is equally important for you. A well-written job description needs to be created and written for each job just once; after that, it merely needs to be occasionally updated. For anyone with access to a computer's word processor, the occasional updating of a disk-stored job description is especially easy.

Operating with a well-written, comprehensive job description has several advantages over not bothering to create one and attempting to carry all of these details in your head:

1) The written description enables you -- the recipient of services -- to have a global, comprehensive reference of your needs for assistance, the schedule of time required to assist those needs, the qualifications of the PCA employees whom you will be hiring, and an objective description of the nature of the work.

2) The written description assures the PCA applicant of an accurate portrayal of the work required as well as the expectations which you have for the type and quality of employee you are willing to hire. This consequently gives you a reference that you can later quote if problems occur with the PCA's job performance.

3) The written description enables you to easily convey details to the PCA applicant during an interview, and thus it minimizes your anxiety during the interview and allows you to observe more about the applicant who is sitting in front of you.

4) The written description enables the applicant to visually examine and better understand the nature and duties of the work, and consequently to make a more informed decision about whether they qualify for and want the job.

5) The written description enhances your image to the applicant being interviewed as a well-organized, authoritative, intelligent individual who should be respected and who can efficiently manage the PCAs and the assistance which they provide.

Parts of a Job Description

There are at least six standard sections to a comprehensive job description, as written for a PCA-type position:

1) Job Title. Although this is usually called a job title, it is often also the title of the employee. The title should identify the type of work to be done. Examples of titles which you might be using include Nurse, Nursing Assistant, Home Health Aide, Personal Care Attendant/Aide, Companion,

Homemaker, Household Maintenance, Housekeeper, Transportation Driver, and Domestic Cook.

2) Nature of Work. This section usually consists of a paragraph or two which introduces the job applicant to the type of work to be done. Topics can include:

■ An introductory (brief) description of the employer and his physical limitations with which the PCA will be working,

■ A brief outline of the type of work required (more detailed information will be provided in the job description section "Duties to be Performed," and

■ A brief outline of the schedule of work required (more detailed information will be provided in the job description section "Duties to be performed."

3) Qualifications and Qualities of Employee. Here you first state whether you require the employee to have formal licensure, certification, training, or experience. The qualifications which you require will vary according to the type of position, since licensure would be expected for some but does not exist for others.

The qualities which you require can include the following:

■ To be dependable, by arriving for work as scheduled or by calling as much in advance as possible when unable to work

■ To be punctual, in meeting the scheduled arrival time or by calling as much in advance as possible when arrival will be delayed by 10 minutes or more

■ To respect the individual to whom assistance is provided, as someone who, regardless of sickness or physical limitations, deserves human respect and a high quality of assistance

■ To respect the individual's confidentiality and privacy regarding their thoughts, values, beliefs, relationships, and activities

- To respect the individual's need for honesty and security, regarding their living quarters, personal possessions, and financial assets

- To maintain a reasonably clean and neat personal appearance, while providing assistance to the individual

- To never arrive for work, or attempt to work, under the negative influence of alcohol, medications, or drugs

- To be willing to discuss and resolve employment-related problems with the employer, and to provide the employer as much advance notice as possible when resigning in order to facilitate finding a replacement

More detail about qualities is included in the chapters "Rights for You and the PCA", "The Top 10 Reasons Why PCAs Quit & Are Fired," and "Job Expectations."

4) Duties to be Performed. This is either your master list of needs for assistance, which you created earlier (see the chapter "Making a Master List of Needs for Assistance"), or a listing created specially for a particular job. In either case, this chart or listing includes the title of each need or group of similar needs, the approximate length of time that need requires, the frequency with which each need occurs, and the approximate starting and stopping times.

> Invite each PCA prospect to take home a copy of your job description, read it, and list any questions that occur to them -- make sure they are comfortable with the duties <u>before</u> they start working

For the job description, you may decide to include your complete master list of needs or just part of it. If a particular job applicant will be performing only a section of this list, because you are dividing duties, then verbally refer the applicant to the appropriate section during the interview.

To include the complete master list, instead of just a partial one, has 2 advantages. First, each applicant gets a global, comprehensive idea of your needs and how their section of work fits into the whole picture. Second, by including the entire master list in the job description, the same job description can be used for all applicants who perform any section of the entire list of duties, and a specialized job description need not be written for each applicant. Of course a different master list should be used for dissimilar jobs, such as medical PCAs and Transportation Drivers.

5) Work Schedule and Comments. This is a summary statement which clarifies the specific days and times for which you expect each employee to arrive and depart.

This "work schedule" section should also mention the procedure you use for making special requests for nonroutine duties, as well as the minimum advance notice you require for the employee to request vacation time or to file a resignation. The minimum advance notice requirements are important to you for lead time in recruiting and scheduling employee fill-ins during vacation periods, or replacements in response to resignations.

6) Salary. This is another standard section of every job description, however a specific salary figure is not always printed. If you expect to be interviewing PCA applicants with a wide range of qualifications and experience, and you will be consequently offering an hourly salary appropriate to these factors, then you may wish to state something like "Salary commensurate with qualifications and experience." However, if you are offering just one specific rate, you may wish to put it in writing in order to attract applicants.

This section should provide as many specifics as desired regarding how the salary is computed, the rate of pay, the pay source, whether benefits are included, and the schedule which you or the 3rd-party funding source uses for issuing paychecks.

Job Description Examples

The purpose of the following job descriptions is to enable you to organize and schedule your PCA needs. This will help you analyze the amount of work you need and enable you to become a more effective PCA manager. The chapter

"Methods for Recruiting PCAs" will concentrate on writing more brief job descriptions for recruiting and advertising.

Here are three examples of job descriptions. The first, brief description illustrates a position for a Transportation Driver; the second and third, longer descriptions apply to the more complex position of a Personal Care Attendant/Aide (PCA).

Job Description

Job Title: Transportation Driver

Nature of the Work:
Marge Janda, who uses motorized wheelchair mobility, works weekdays as a computer programmer at the Saratoga Access & Fitness Company. While she owns a lift-equipped van, she does not drive and needs someone to drive her between her home and work site. The round-trip distance is 24 miles. The transportation driver is asked to arrive at Marge's house each weekday morning, drive her to work, and drive the empty van back to her house. The driver is then on his own time during the day until the driving cycle is repeated in late afternoon in order to transport her back home.

Qualifications and Quality of Employee:
The Transportation Driver must have a valid driver's license and is asked to observe the following qualities toward Marge and the work:

■ To be dependable, by arriving for work as scheduled or by calling as much in advance as possible when unable to work

■ To be punctual, in meeting the scheduled arrival time or by calling as much in advance as possible when arrival will be delayed by 10 minutes or more

■ To respect Marge as someone who, regardless of sickness or physical limitations, deserves human respect and a high quality of assistance

■ To respect Marge's confidentiality and privacy regarding her thoughts, values, beliefs, relationships, and activities

Creating a Job Description for PCAs

■ To respect Marge's need for honesty and security, regarding her living quarters, personal possessions, and financial assets

■ To maintain a reasonably clean and neat personal appearance, while providing assistance to Marge

■ To never arrive at work, or attempt to work, under the negative influence of alcohol, medications, or drugs

■ To be willing to discuss and resolve employment-related problems with Marge, and to provide her as much advance notice as possible when resigning in order to facilitate finding a replacement

Duties to be Performed:
a) Arrive at Marge's home by 8:00 am on each weekday morning for which she is working,
b) Come inside, assist her with any outdoor clothing, and help her get to and into the van,
c) Drive her the 12 miles to work which takes approximately 25 minutes in morning traffic,
d) Provide any necessary assistance from her van into her job site,
e) Return the empty van to her home driveway,
f) Arrive at her home by 4:30 pm and drive the empty van to her job site for a 5 pm pickup, and
g) Drive Marge home.

> Be complete in listing all of your needs for assistance; don't hide the more unpleasant ones to make the job seem more attractive to prospects

Work Schedule and Comments:
Assistance is needed in the morning and afternoon of each weekday that Marge works. She may make special trip requests in as much advance as possible to determine whether the driver can accommodate them. It will be assumed that the driver will not be making personal side trips with the empty van unless permission is obtained fror Marge. In addition, if Marge would like occasional "er van" errands performed by the driver while she is a⁺ she will make these requests in as much ad·

possible. The driver is asked to provide at least a 2-week advance notice for vacation time and a 4-week notice for resignation in order to enable Marge to find replacement help.

Salary:
The hourly salary is paid for the average round trip time the driver spends on the road, from the time of arrival at the house to dropping off the empty van. These times average 8-9:30 am and 4:30-6 pm and will be the basis for a 3-hour pay period each day unless significant exceptions occur. The hourly rate is $5.00 and is paid personally by Marge; paychecks are issued each Friday afternoon unless requested for another time. All standard salary taxes are withheld; no benefits or paid vacation/sick time are provided.

Job Description

Job Title: Personal Care Aide/Attendant (PCA), part-time

Nature of Work:
Suzy Rose is a college student at the State University. A recent car accident caused a spinal cord injury and resulted in paralysis and a loss of sensation below chest level. In addition, she has a partial use of her arms and wrists. She uses a motorized wheelchair and drives a lift-equipped van. While attending SU for pre-law studies, she needs a PCA who is also her campus dorm roommate. She needs assistance in the morning and at night, and she is usually independent in activities throughout the day and during on- and off-campus social activities.

College students who need PCA help usually find that other students are very willing to earn extra money by providing assistance...as either PCA-roommates or as PCAs who are met at specified campus locations during the day

Creating a Job Description for PCAs 237

Qualifications and Quality of Employee:
Trained and experienced personal care attendants/aides are welcome to apply, however student applicants with no experience are welcome if they have the following qualities:

- To be dependable, by arriving for work as scheduled or by calling as much in advance as possible when unable to work

- To be punctual, in meeting the scheduled arrival time or by calling as much in advance as possible when arrival will be delayed by 10 minutes or more

- For the PCA roommate who shares Suzy's dorm room to be always present in the room whenever Suzy is in bed, due to Suzy's inability to independently get out of bed or attend to sudden medical or personal needs in an emergency

- To respect Suzy as someone who, regardless of sickness or physical limitations, deserves human respect and a high quality of assistance

- To respect Suzy's confidentiality and privacy regarding her thoughts, values, beliefs, relationships, and activities

- To respect Suzy's need for honesty and security, regarding her living quarters, personal possessions, and financial assets

- To maintain a reasonably clean and neat personal appearance, while providing assistance to Suzy

- To never arrive at work, or attempt to work, under the negative influence of alcohol, medications, or drugs

- To be willing to discuss and resolve employment-related problems with Suzy, and to provide her as much advance notice as possible when resigning in order to facilitate finding a replacement

Duties to be Performed:
Each part-time PCA will be asked to perform a specific section of Suzy's master list of needs shown below. That

section will be identified and discussed at the on-site interview with Suzy or her PCA Coordinator.

Master List of Needs for Assistance
[Editorial note to readers: For illustrative purposes, examples of both male and female needs for assistance are provided in the following list.]

Title of Need	How Long	Frequency	Approx Start/Stop Times
■ morning meds in bed	2 min	each morn	7 am
■ empty bladder	2 min	each morn	
■ change/clean urinary device	10 min	each morn	7:05-7:15
■ begin dressing in bed: socks, binder, underware	10 min	each morn	7:15-7.25
■ transfer to wheelchair & adjust position	5 min	each morn	7:25-7:30
■ wash & groom at sink	20 min	each morn	7:30-7:50
■finish dressing from waist up	5 min	each morn	7:50-7:55
■ Suzy leaves the college dorm room for breakfast in the cafeteria & will continue on to the day's classes and activities		each day	8:00 am+

Creating a Job Description for PCAs 239

■ meet a PCA or cafeteria staff for help:
go thru line, get food, carry tray to table, prepare food — 10 min — each day — 8am b'fast; 12n lunch; 5pm dinner

■ meet a PCA in a restroom to assist legbag empty/ feminine hygiene/ catheter bladder empty — 10 min — each day — 10am,12n, 2pm,4pm

■ laundry — 3 hrs — M-Th eves & after accidents — after 7pm

■ clean bedroom & bath floors, clean bathroom sinks-mirror-toilet-shower, change bedsheets — 45 min — M-Th eves during laundry — after 7pm

■ water plants — 20 min — M-W-F eves — after 7 pm

■ bowel/douche routine & shower — 1.5 hrs — Su-T-Th eves — 7:30-9:00pm

■ help into bed: wash at sink, eve meds, transfer to bed, undress, & position — 25 min — each night — 10-10:25pm

■ bowel or bladder accident cleanup — 1 hr ave — unpredictable

- clean wheelchair, check battery levels   20 min   once/week after dinner
- repair wheelchr   varies   unpredictable
- wash & wax van   3 hrs   spring & fall

Work Schedule and Comments:
The specific schedule of duties will be identified and discussed at the on-site interview. In addition to the listed duties, the PCA will be occasionally asked to assist with nonroutine duties. These will be requested and scheduled in as much advance as possible with the PCA. Due to the continuous dependence of Suzy on assistance, PCAs are requested to provide at least a week's advance notice of desired vacation time and a 4-week notice of intention to resign. These advance notices are important for scheduling vacation fill-in help, or for recruiting replacements for resigning help.

Salary:
The starting salary range is $4.25-$5.50 per hour, depending upon previous training and experience of applicant. Satisfactory job performance will be rewarded with a $.25 per hour merit increase after 3 months of steady employment and on each 3-month anniversary of the starting date. No health insurance benefits or paid vacation/sick time are included. Suzy pays salaries from personal funds and paychecks will be issued each week on a standard day to be determined during the on-site interview.

Job Description

Job Title: Personal Care Aide/Attendant (PCA), part-time

Nature of Work:
Tyrone Gossett, age 56, is recuperating at home for an undeterminable period of time after hospital discharge from a stroke. He is attempting to gradually return to work during these later stages of recuperation. The left-side CVA has resulted in paralysis to the right half of his body, impaired speech, and partial incontinence of bowel and bladder. Tyrone needs several hours of daily assistance which he has chosen to divide among several part-time aides in order to minimize the negative effects of any aide's

Creating a Job Description for PCAs

inability to work. Types of assistance include changing and cleaning of urinary incontinence devices, dressing, transfers between bed and wheelchair, grooming, showering, toileting, cooking, feeding, laundry, and household chores.

Qualifications and Quality of Employee:
Trained and experienced personal care aides/attendants/nursing assistants are welcome to apply, however applicants with no experience will be considered if they have the following qualities:

■ To be dependable, by arriving for work as scheduled or by calling as much in advance as possible when unable to work

■ To be punctual, in meeting the scheduled arrival time or by calling as much in advance as possible when arrival will be delayed by 10 minutes or more

■ To respect Tyrone as someone who, regardless of sickness or physical limitations, deserves human respect and a high quality of assistance

■ To respect Tyrone's confidentiality and privacy regarding his thoughts, values, beliefs, relationships, and activities

■ To respect Tyrone's need for honesty and security, regarding his living quarters, personal possessions, and financial assets

■ To maintain a reasonably clean and neat personal appearance, while providing assistance to Tyrone

■ To never arrive at work, or attempt to work, under the negative influence of alcohol, medications, or drugs

■ To be willing to discuss and resolve employment-related problems with Tyrone, and to provide him as much advance notice as possible when resigning in order to facilitate finding a replacement

Duties to be Performed:
Each part-time PCA will be asked to perform a specific section of the master list of needs shown below. That section will be identified and discussed at the on-site interview with Mr. Gossett or his PCA Coordinator.

Master List of Needs for Assistance
[Editorial note to readers: For illustrative purposes, examples of both male and female needs for assistance are provided in the following list.]

Title of Need	How Long	Frequency	Approx Start/ Stop Times
∎ morning meds in bed	2 min	each morn	7 am
∎ empty bladder	2 min	each morn	
∎ change urinary device	10 min	each morn	7:05-7:15
∎ begin dressing in bed: socks, binder, underware	10 min	each morn	7:15-7.25
∎ transfer to wheelchair & adjust position	5 min	each morn	7:25-7:30
∎ wash & groom at sink	20 min	each morn	7:30-7:50
∎finish dressing from waist up	5 min	each morn	7:50-7:55
∎ cook breakfast, eat, put dishes into d'washer	20 min	each morn	8:00-8:20
∎ dress for outside & transfer to car	10 min	each wkday	8:20-8:30

Creating a Job Description for PCAs 243

- commute to work with driver — 20 min — each wkday 8:30-8:50

- at work: transfer from car to wheelchair & go to worksite — 10 min — each wkday 8:50-9:00

- meet a PCA to empty legbag in a restroom — 10 min — each wkday 10am,12n, 2pm,4pm

- meet a PCA or cafeteria staff for lunchroom help: go thru line, get food, carry tray to table, prepare food, eat — 45 min — each wkday 11a-12:30p

- meet a PCA at home for lunch: cook, serve food, eat — 45 min — each nonworkdy 11a-12:30p

- dress for outside & transfer to car — 10 min — each wkday 5-5:10pm

- commute to home with driver — 30 min — each wkday 5:15-5:45

- transfer from car — 10 min — each wkday 5:50-6:00

- cook dinner, serve food, eat, dishes into d'washer — 60 min — each eve 6:00-7:00

- grocery shop — 2 hrs — Fri eves 7:15-9:15p

- laundry — 3 hrs — M-Th eves & after accidents after 7pm

- mop kitchen &
bath floors, vacuum,
bedroom & living
room, clean
bathroom sinks-
mirror-toilet-shower,
change bedsheets   45 min   M-Th eves
                                      during
                                      laundry   after 7pm

- water plants   20 min   M-W-F eves after 7 pm

- bowel/douche
routine & shower   1.5 hrs   Su-T-Th
                                      eves   7:30-9:00p

- help into bed:
wash at sink, eve
meds, transfer to
bed, undress, &
position   25 min   each night 10-10:25p

- bowel or bladder
accident cleanup   1 hr ave   unpredictable

- clean wheelchair,
check battery levels   20 min   once/week   after dinner

- repair wheelchr   varies   unpredictable

- defrost kitchen
freezer   20 min   spring & fall

- wash & wax car   3 hrs   spring & fall

- wash apartment
windows   2 hrs   spring & fall

Work Schedule and Comments:
The specific schedule of duties will be identified and discussed at the on-site interview. In addition to the listed duties, the PCA will be occasionally asked to assist with nonroutine duties. These will be advance requested and scheduled with the PCA whenever possible. Due to the

continuous dependence of Mr. Gossett on assistance, PCAs are requested to provide at least a week's advance notice of desired vacation time and a 4-week notice of intention to resign. These advance notices are important for scheduling vacation fill-in help, or for recruiting replacements for resigning help.

Salary:
The starting salary range is $4.25-$5.50 per hour, depending upon previous training and experience of an applicant. Satisfactory job performance will be rewarded with a $.25 per hour merit increase after 3 months of steady employment and on each 6-month anniversary of the starting date. No health insurance benefits or paid vacation/sick time are included. Mr. Gossett pays salaries from county-supplied funds and paychecks will be issued each 2 weeks on a standard day to be determined by the county.

23. Residence Locations for a PCA

The PCAs you hire might live a considerable distance from your residence, quite closeby, or in fact, might share your residence with you. It is important to be familiar with the advantages and disadvantages of the distance between your living locations as well as whether one or two PCAs should live with you. The details of this section will give you strategies for:

a) Improving the chances that a PCA will maintain a dependable record of coming to work,

b) Improving the chances that a PCA will punctually arrive on schedule and have less of a desire to leave early,

c) Improving the chances that a PCA will want to keep the job for a long period of time,

d) Saving you out-of-pocket money, and decreasing your personal income taxes and tax paperwork, by substituting live-in (noncash) job benefits for part or all of a cash salary, and

e) Increasing the availability of PCA assistance while safeguarding your current privacy and security of personal possessions.

> A live-in PCA is essential for many folks who cannot independently transfer out of bed in an emergency or take care of certain personal or medical needs that may suddenly occur...and yes, roommates can be changed when they no longer want to be PCAs

There are 5 primary residence options for any PCA. Each has advantages and disadvantages which you should consider. You might decide to offer or even require one or more of the PCAs who work for you to take up one of the live-in options. If you do not wish to involve yourself with a live-in option, you should be aware of the residence distance from you to each of the PCA prospects whom you are considering for hire. For some suburban or rural settings discussed below, a considerable distance will not present a deterrent for your hiring a PCA; for other, heavily-populated city situations, a prospect who lives only a few blocks away might be a poor risk for hiring. The following are categories of options which relate your living situation to each PCA.

1) Live-in option: One or more PCAs as your roommate

>   The setting for using this option is usually a college campus dorm room or a one-bedroom apartment, condo, or house. You and the PCA(s) who works for you share a bedroom as roommates. Some folks have found that bunk beds in a college dorm room even make it possible to have more than one PCA roommate.
>
>   The advantages of this PCA residence option are at least 3-fold. First, there is usually readily available assistance when urgent and unscheduled needs arise, when turning during the night is necessary, or if a fire or medical emergency suddenly occurs. Second, there is seldom a problem with "no shows" of a PCA not arriving on schedule in the morning, unless the PCA decides to leave your room and sleep elsewhere. Third, this option can be used for offering a noncash-salary benefit to the PCA. This last advantage is discussed in more detail in the chapter, "Types of Monetary Salaries: Cash, Noncash, & Both."
>
>   The primary disadvantage to you and the PCA is a lack of privacy, quiet, and living space. As a group, you and your roommates are constantly sharing your living and sleeping space. Numerous compromises and sacrifices will be necessary in order to maintain smooth living relations. In addition, with PCA help usually readily available, you must be very careful to resist the temptation of asking for instant assistance whenever the slightest need arises. The PCA and you do live in the same quarters, however -- for the PCA's sanity -- this cannot mean that the PCA is "on duty" and a "butler-in-waiting" for whenever you might need something. Write out your Master List of Needs and stick to requesting assistance only during the times listed unless a really urgent, unscheduled need arises. Otherwise, you will quickly burn out and lose the PCA. More details on when to and

when not to ask for help are found in the chapters, "Abusing Help with Inappropriate Requests" and "3 Types of Activities Which Qualify for PCA Help."

2) Live-in option: The PCA(s) lives in the same living area, but has a sleeping room separate from yours

For this setting, the PCA(s) sleeps in a part of the same college dormitory suite, apartment, condo, or house which is separate from your sleeping area. For example, if you have a 2-bedroom apartment, you could occupy one bedroom by yourself and offer the 2nd bedroom to be shared by one or two PCAs who are students at a nearby college. As a group, you share the bathroom(s), kitchen, and livingroom.

The advantages and disadvantages are much the same as those of the first option, except that everyone has a bit more privacy, quiet, and living space -- especially you!

3) Live-nearby option: The PCA(s) lives in the same building, but in a separate college dorm room, apartment, or condo

For this setting, you and the PCA have the privacy of separate living quarters. For example, the setting might be a college campus residence hall with 75 student dorm rooms or an apartment complex with 75 apartments. You occupy one of these rooms or apartments and one or more PCAs who work for you live separately or together in their own room or apartment within the same building. You can readily communicate with each other by telephone (wired or cordless), wireless intercom, pager, or any of the other innovative devices which are inexpensively featured at Radio Shack-type stores.

> An overall rule-of-thumb: the greater the distance between your residence and a PCA's, the greater the chance for no-shows, late arrivals, & the PCA quickly tiring of commuting to the job

The advantages include increased privacy and living space for both parties over sharing the same quarters. The PCA is far enough away to provide this privacy, however close enough to provide assistance for urgent, unscheduled needs for help.

Good communication is the key to the success for this closeby-but-separated setting. The 2 important communication elements are a well-defined work schedule, drawn from your Master List of Needs, and probably an adequate electronic communication system. This telephone, intercom, or pager system should have at least one station within your reach while you are in bed. The device is essential if, during the night when you are alone in bed, an urgent and unscheduled personal need for assistance occurs, a fire or medical emergency arises, or the PCA does not "arise" on time in the morning.

The primary disadvantage is the probability of unavailable assistance when the 2-element communication system is not adequate...that is if PCAs do not have a clear work schedule of when each is to assist you, or if there is no way for you to quickly contact the PCA living quarters when a sudden problem occurs.

4) Live-nearby option: The PCA(s) live nearby in the same neighborhood, or in a reasonable distance within the same or a nearby town

For this setting, you have your own private residence and the PCAs have theirs. They could live within a block or so of your residence, or several miles away in the next town.

The primary advantage is the maximum privacy and amount of living space for you, and possibly your family members who live with you.

The primary disadvantage is the increasing chance for the PCA to "no show" or to often arrive significantly late for scheduled work. In addition, if you live alone and without family members, there is the increased chance that occasional, urgent needs will be unassisted because a PCA will be unable or unwilling to travel to your residence when you phone with an urgent, unscheduled need for assistance.

Consequently, with each increase in distance between you and the PCAs, there is an increase in the wisdom of having several backup PCAs. This can mean dividing your needs with more than one part-time PCA, and keeping everyone's phone number handy by your bedside for the occasion that a scheduled PCA is suddenly unable to work.

The potential for PCA problems is linked to both the geographical distance between your residence and the PCA's, as well as the number of people who live, work, or travel within that distance. If you live in a less populated suburban, country, or rural area, then a 5-mile distance between you and the PCA would probably not present a deterrent to the PCA arriving as scheduled. However, if you live in a very densely populated city full of traffic, subways, buses, trolleys, and muggers, then a 5-block commute might often result in considerable fatigue, hassle, and time as deterrents for the PCA to arrive punctually...or, sometimes, at all!

5) Combination option: You employ more than one PCA and combine the use of live-in and live-nearby PCAs

With the combo approach, you hire more than one PCA for the advantages discussed in the chapter "Dividing Needs With More Than One PCA." In hiring PCAs, you might hire one or two live-ins in addition to others who live nearby. Including at least one live-in PCA is particularly wise for those who live alone and are dependent upon assistance for urgent, unscheduled needs or for evacuation help during a fire or sudden medical emergency. If, on the other hand, you live with family members, you will probably choose to hire PCAs who live nearby.

In summary, different residence options exist and you should assess which is best for your own needs, your desire for privacy, your need for physical help during night-time emergencies, and the availability of PCAs in your comunity.

24. Sources for Recruiting PCAs

In any community, several sources exist for finding people who are willing to provide PCA assistance. Some of these people will have considerable experience. Others will have no experience and must be both oriented to the personal nature of the work, so they feel comfortable, and then be trained, so they perform duties according to the safe and efficient methods you prefer.

Below is a listing of the most common sources for targeting your recruiting. It should not be viewed as an exhaustive list, since you will probably develop additional sources particular to your living situation and its community.

> There are at least 8 common sources to tap for finding PCAs in most communities -- your locale might have unique sources of its own

1) Referrals from Current PCAs

When a current PCA announces to you that she wishes to take vacation time or to resign, she and other PCAs represent the first step to finding either temporary fill-in help or a longer-term replacement.

If the two of you have maintained a relationship of mutual respect, your current PCA will usually be quite willing to consult her personal contacts for possible new assistance. If your employment relationship is ending on a sour note, then your current PCA will not usually be very interested in helping you with your recruiting efforts.

Your request of your current PCA is simple...to ask whether she knows of any friends or PCA colleagues who might be looking for work. The next stage is to ask for her suggestions and ideas about general sources for recruiting by you in the area community.

2) Previous PCA applicants or PCA employees

Before spending effort, time, and possibly money on recruiting new PCAs from scratch, be sure that all currently known resources have been used.

To further illustrate this strategy, think of the last time you were grocery shopping. If you thought that you might need certain food items, you undoubtedly checked your own refrigerator and pantry for any existing supply of these items before you ran to the store to purchase new amounts. After all, it is commonsense not to waste effort, time, and money on buying something new if you still have a usable, former supply of the same thing. The same logic applies to hiring PCAs.

When you last recruited PCAs, you should have kept a listing of the applicants who were fully qualified and desirable, but who were not hired. For example, at the last time that you recruited, perhaps you received applications from 8 potential PCAs. During the interviews, you eliminated 3 undesirables. Maybe 1 additional applicant failed to show up for his appointment visit to see your routine. Since you needed 2 PCAs at that time, you hired the 2 applicants who were the most desirable, leaving 2 more applicants who were also fully qualified. Hopefully, you didn't toss out the information about these second-stringers, but you kept the details about them for possible future use.

Now, you need additional PCAs; now is the time to call the second-stringers to ask if they are still interested in working for you. In some cases, previous PCAs (whose work was satisfactory) might be willing to resume working for you. If so, no additional recruiting is necessary. Further details are included in the chapter "Interviewing, Screening, and Hiring Prospective PCAs."

3) Home health aide agency

If you are unable or unwilling to recruit PCAs on your own, requesting already employed aides from an agency is essential. On the other hand, even if you do plan to recruit on your own, agency employed aides are handy when:

a) You are new to a community and as yet unaware of the potential sources of PCAs within your new locale,

b) Your personal recruiting for some reason is not resulting in a sufficient number of applications, or

c) You have an urgent need for new PCA help in the next few hours, and this urgency prevents taking the few days of time which personal recruiting often requires.

If you do wish to recruit and manage PCAs whom you directly employ, but you find yourself in one of these three situations, you might decide to request agency aides for a temporary period of time until you are successful in your own recruiting. Just be careful not to sign any contract with the home health agency for a period of time beyond the date that you believe your personal recruiting will be successful. The advantages of your directly employing PCAs, instead of using agency aides, have been detailed previously in this handbook, and they begin with savings in hourly salary rates (when you pay salaries from your own pocket) as well as increased management control.

4) Nearby college campus

College students have several qualities that make some of them excellent PCA prospects. They are young, physically fit, strong, and healthy. Their personal schedules are flexible because of a lack of local family life and they have few time commitments beyond classes, meals, studying, extracurricular activities and sports, and romantic experimentations. Perhaps most importantly, most college students either need money or think they do.

On the down side, some students have tendencies to be immature in not being punctual or reliable, and in quickly dismissing responsibilities for study time for upcoming exams and papers, for higher paying and easier jobs, or for satisfying their sexual libidos. Consequently, a college student's punctuality, reliability, and overall responsibility are considerably increased when they live either in a live-in situation or very close to you.

The 18 to 22 year age of undergraduate students is also a factor to be discussed. Students are most successfully used when the difference between their age and yours is minimal. For, as the difference increases, you -- the senior -- more and more resemble the parents from whom the student is seeking emotional independence. You become a "grown up" who should be addressed by a title and last name, such as "Mr. Breu" or "Mrs. Santiago" instead of "Terry" or "Debbie." With each succeeding year, the typical 20 year old is less comfortable in providing you with very personal, physical assistance unless perhaps they have a tendency toward a medical career. As one college female once said, "I'm 19 years old and Mr. Littlefield is 42. Helping him get dressed would be like helping one of my father's buddies put on his pants...it would make me feel kind of odd." Non-personal chores, however, such as housecleaning, lawn work, transportation, or house painting, are much less vulnerable to age differences.

Additionally, as you become older, you are less likely to be patient with a sporadic lack of punctuality, reliability, or responsibility. In short, up to your age of about 35, using college students can be very successful. Beyond 35, you may find yourself seeking older, more mature, more stable sources of PCAs. In any case, it is wise to favor upperclassmen (juniors and seniors) and graduate students over first-year freshmen and second-year sophomores, even though the eager and energetic freshmen and sophomores will often be the first respondents to PCA ads which you posted in a campus area. The eager freshman often doesn't yet have a realistic sense of time demands for college life, whereas the upperclassman often has worked out a study routine and can make commitments with more reliability. Using high school students is rarely recommended.

> College students, regardless of their lack of PCA experience, often make ideal PCAs for younger folks who need assistance & who have good management skills

Although college students can be recruited at almost anytime, there are some notably good and bad recruiting times at any typical college campus. Good times include the beginning of any semester, before academic responsibilities start to pile up and while students are still rested from vacations. Logically then, bad times to recruit are most likely to be during the last 3 or 4 weeks of a semester, when exams, term papers, romantic pursuits, and other sources of fatigue are overwhelming most student desires for taking on new responsibilities. Some students, however, are willing at the end of one semester to commit themselves to a job which will start with the beginning of the next semester...a fact which is very important to consider for advance recruiting for continuous PCA needs.

The schedule of when semesters begin and end varies among colleges, however the details are readily available by calling the campus.

If you live on or nearby a college campus, there are several routes for finding interested and quite capable students to supply different categories of PCA help:

a) Many colleges have established a professional, administrative office which exists to advise and serve special needs of campus members with various disabilities. Popular titles include Disabled Student Services, Disability Services, Rehabilitation Services, and Handicapped Student Center. Professional staff at this department or office can be tapped for information about PCA recruiting markets, recruiting methods, popular hourly salaries, and formal PCA programs (on campuses where they exist).

b) The student newspaper at the campus is often the best way of advertising a PCA job with students. Most campuses host a student paper, and the paper almost always welcomes paid classified and display ads of any kind regardless of whether the source originates on or off campus. A phone call to the paper's office can get prices, and ads can often be placed over the phone when payment is made by credit card number or a bill is sent to you. There is more detail on writing, designing, and placing newspaper ads in a the later chapter "Methods for Recruiting PCAs."

c) Bulletin and notice boards on a campus are usually spread throughout residence halls (dormitories), dining halls (cafeterias), academic buildings, and administrative buildings. Many of these cork boards have clearly printed limitations regarding the subject matter and size of notices that can be posted; violating notices are often torn down.

Campus buildings are usually open to the public with the exceptions of dining halls during mealtimes or residence halls, libraries, and some classroom areas which require each entering individual too show a campus ID card for purposes of building security. You may wish to take a walk through some of the primary campus buildings to "case out" the locations of bulletin boards and the type of notices displayed. With this advance information, make up your posters or notice cards of an appropriate type and size and then return to the campus to put them in strategic places for maximum visibility. More detail on composing and strategically posting notices is found in the later chapter "Methods for Recruiting PCAs."

d) The student employment office of most campuses assists students in finding part-time jobs while they are students. This office is different from the career planning/placement office, which assists students with post-college careers for the future, or the personnel office, which assists the college in recruiting faculty and staff for its own professional employment needs. The student employment office will often accept job announcements from both on and off campus employers. These announcements are usually posted on notice boards or filed in job notebooks which job-seeking students browse through each day. You should feel free to call a campus student employment office to inquire about their announcing your PCA job.

e) The campus personnel office, while not usually providing a way of reaching students, might be willing to post your notice for older, non-student folks to see. Give them a call to inquire about whether the personnel office exists to promote only jobs offered by the college institution or whether it will post to its employees the chance for the extra "moonlighting" work offered by your PCA job.

f) Student clubs and organizations are usually numerous at any campus. It may take some inquiry from insiders, but locating certain types of student clubs can be sometimes very useful in spreading the word about your PCA needs. Specific kinds of student groups might be of particular interest to you. Groups which gather students with a medical concentration might be centered around academic majors in physical therapy, occupational therapy, rehabilitation counseling, nursing, or pre med. Students with such academic interests can be especially good candidates for PCA jobs.

You can often locate such groups -- if indeed these or similar medical fields are offered at the particular campus -- by calling or visiting the student program office which coordinates and supervises all student clubs, by finding students who are members of a desired club, by consulting with the faculty advisor to such a club, or by contacting the actual office headquarters for the organization. Inquire about posting your job notice in that office or having a member read out your notice at the club's next meeting.

5) Surrounding community

The community around you contains several categories of people who will probably be interested in PCA work. Perhaps the primary categories are aides who --

- are already employed in a local hospital or by home health aide agencies, and who desire extra money with a "moonlighting" job, or

- are not employed by institutions or agencies because they prefer the self-employment freedom of directly contracting their services to private individuals.

Other categories of folks who might be interested in PCA work include people from non-medical fields; college students, retired folks, and friends who already know you; and finally weirdos of several shapes and kinds who should be avoided.

More details about creating and placing ads are found in the chapter "Methods for Recruiting PCAs"; details about identifying, weeding out, and avoiding the weirdos is included in "Interviewing, Screening, and Hiring Prospective PCAs."

> "Moonlighting aides" who are looking for part-time work beyond their regular jobs can often be found by placing newspaper ads or by checking aide listings which are available to the public from local medical facilities

The categories include those with medical training who have considerable experience in performing PCA-like duties, as well as those who have no experience in this area but who are interested in earning extra money by assisting someone.

The most desirable type, of course, is the individual with related experience. The advantage of this experience is not so much their training in medical procedures, but their basic awareness of the personal nature of the work and their degree of comfort with that work. Remember though, that regardless of someone's medical training or previous experience, they will still depend on your instructions and management skills in determining which specific duties you require -- and how you prefer those duties performed.

For many of us who especially wish to find "moonlighting aides," tapping the surrounding community can be the most fruitful way of finding PCA help. An ad in the local newspaper is usually the most cost effective and least laborious way to reach the greatest number of people in the community. Posters in supermarkets and shopping malls have been known to produce limited results, however the newspaper ad is by far the most productive.

6) Local medical facility

Local medical facilities may have home health aide listings or they may provide a source for posting notices. Such community medical facilities can include a hospital, rehabilitation center, nursing home, HMO (health maintenance organization), clinic, or ambulance corps (commercial or volunteer).

Certain types of medical facilities, such as hospitals and public health departments, often maintain listings of home health aide agencies as well as private aides. These lists are used mainly by patients being discharged who will require assistance at home, however hospitals are often willing to share these lists with anyone who needs assistance. If a facility does maintain lists of agencies or private aides, the lists are typically available from the facility's Office of Discharge Planning, Social Work, or similar department.

Contacting the staff of the medical facility may also yield results. The objective is to inform the institution's staff of the PCA position you are offering in case anyone desires some spare-time work.

Some institutions are quite protective of "their" staff and will not permit notices of "competing" jobs. The institutions fear that staff members who work extra jobs will show the effects of fatigue or a decreasing interest in their jobs at the institution. Consequently, the posting of notices within the institution to medical staff usually requires either the permission of the administration or the advice and help of one of the staff who will know both whether notices are appropriate and where to post them for you.

7) Disability organizations in a campus or community

Disability organizations can include independent living programs, state or city offices for those with handicaps or disabilities, a college campus administrative office or student organization, and area or local citizen groups.

In any event, these groups might be handy for your personal recruiting efforts for at least two categories of information. First, they can advise you about the PCA market in your living area, including where and how to recruit along with the popular hourly salary rates being paid to PCAs. The organization might even have established a PCA pool of folks who have registered with the organization because of interest in being employed as PCAs.

Second, the group might publish a periodic newsletter and therefore be willing to include your PCA notice. The trick in using newsletters is to hope that a monthly or bimonthly newsletter will be printed and promptly distributed within the time that you are recruiting a PCA. That schedule matchup is often very difficult to accomplish.

In any event, your inquiry -- for whatever reason -- with a nearby disability organization will usually result in time and effort well spent. These groups usually have a number of services which will be helpful to you.

8) Employment agency

Many communities have government or commercially operated employment agencies listed in the telephone yellow pages. These agencies function as brokers between people looking for jobs and employers offering jobs. Each agency has its own procedures, so you should feel free to call any area agency to determine whether it can be of assistance for your finding either experienced aides or inexperienced-but-willing-to-learn folks to supply PCA help.

When you call, have a clear, brief, and concise PCA job description ready in case the agency requests it, and ask about who pays any fee which the agency might require for its brokerage services.

In summary, while there are 8 common sources for locating PCAs, there might be other sources in your community. Talking with other people who use PCAs, or with people who work as PCAs, may help you locate any additional sources for recruitiing.

25. Methods for Recruiting PCAs

Some Secrets of Advertising

Picture yourself as an aide or prospective PCA who is searching for a job by looking through the "Help Wanted" ads of today's paper or browsing over posters on a bulletin board. As you scan the many ads, you are glad to find two which offer PCA jobs. Which of these sounds more attractive and friendly? To which one would you apply first?

> Help Handicapped; part-time, must be flexible; state hours available, reasons for wanting job, wage desired, & references. Send resume to: P.O. Box 297, Fonda, NY 12068.

> EARN $80 PER MONTH for just 4 1/2 hours per week; wheelchair male needs help to dress, etc. M-W-F, 7-8:30 am; need now, will train, please call 583-1972.

The much more attractive ad is the second one. That ad will probably receive several responses. The individual who placed the second ad tried to make the ad and the job appealing and attractive to prospective PCAs. The first ad is less appealing, in part, because it doesn't offer the PCA prospect any reason to want the job or to respond to the ad -- sort of like fishing with a bare hook and no bait! The first ad merely demands information from the reader.

The second ad illustrates how to successfully recruit. The strategies which follow apply to most forms of advertising, including newspaper and newsletter ads, posters, and index card notices for bulletin boards.

Before getting into details, let's illustrate a few concepts of marketing and advertising with a story told at a professional seminar for advertising agencies. The lecturer told us about her personal love for chocolate covered ice cream bars.

"I want to tell you how very much I love the taste of ice cream bars with that crunchy chocolate coating. You could get me to attend a dinner even at my in-laws' home if you promised me an ice cream bar for dessert. There are a lot of people like me who have a deep seated passion for those things.

"In my spare time, I like to fish for trout and bass. When I was a kid, I figured that since I loved ice cream bars, the fish would also. I actually tried fishing with one on my hook one time and, of course, didn't attract any fish. Because to attract fish, you have to picture yourself as a fish for a moment and ask yourself 'what food would attract me to risk getting caught on a fisherman's hook.' The answer is worms, and you must use worms to attract a fish regardless of whether worms would appeal to you. The same lesson applies to wording advertisements in order to attract customers to buy a product."

> The golden rule for attracting PCAs to your ads: Determine what desires, wants, or needs the PCAs in your area are most likely to have, and then make sure the salary or benefits of your job satisfy some of those desires

The moral of this story for attracting PCA prospects by advertising is to try to picture the type of person that will apply for your position and to ask yourself what features of the job would appeal to prospects, and therefore attract them to apply to work for you. Once these attractive features are identified, they should be included in newspaper ads, posters, and other notices.

Here's how it is done.

In addition to putting attractive features in the ad and painting a favorable image for the PCA job, there is a successful formula of essential parts for structuring a poster, index card notice, or newspaper ad.

The headline -- the most attractive benefit, or a title which describes the job or a desirable type of applicant
The lead line -- more detail about the attractive benefits
The description of obligations -- what needs to be done?
The sense of urgency -- tell them to apply now
The contact info -- how do they reach you?

■ **The brief, attractive headline.** The objective of the heading, or headline, is to catch the reader's eye and to entice her into reading the rest of the ad or notice. In composing your poster, index card notice, or newspaper ad, the first objective is to catch the eye of prospects who are casually scanning an entire bulletin board full of notices (or the crowded classified ad page of a newspaper). A general, non-specific heading of "Help Wanted," "Job," or "Handicapped Needs Help" will hardly be attractive enough to catch her eye.

Instead, determine some benefits that would attract a prospective PCA to want to provide you with help, and use those benefits in the heading:

    Weekly Salary
    Earn $80 Per Month
    Earn $ Now
    Free Furn Apt
    Free Balcony Apt
    Free Apt & Utils

An alternate approach for a heading is to use a brief title which describes the job or a desirable type of individual:

    Household Help
    Companion to Senior Citizen
    Nursing Student
    Pre-Med Student
    Home Health Aide

These headings and ones similar to them are attention grabbers and spark the prospective PCA's curiosity. Consequently, she steps up to the poster to get a closer look at the details, or to read the rest of the newspaper ad, in order to learn about how to take advantage of the attractive benefits stated in the heading.

∎ **The lead line.** After the large print headline is the lead line. This is usually smaller in print and includes details about additional benefits. Here the reader finds more detail of the sweet deal found in the heading and she further develops interest in the offer. There is purposely no mention yet of any obligation.

Think of this process in terms of attracting fish to a fisherman's hook and line. The brief, large-print heading attracts the PCA much like the fat, juicy, wiggly worm catches the attention of a passing fish. The fish, like the PCA, steps up to the worm to get a better look. The lead line of the poster or ad, just like a closer look at the fresh worm, tells the PCA prospect, "Here's a good sounding deal...keep nibbling...I think you'll like the taste of this deal.'

In each of the examples later, you will find an attention grabbing heading followed by the further explanation of a lead line. Depending upon the amount of message content in the poster, index card notice, or newspaper ad, the lead line section might consist of a single phrase or several sentences.

∎ **The description of obligation.** This section is very brief, and sketches the "what, where, when, and how often" of the duties which must be done in return for receiving the benefits. It should be fair and not sugarcoated, however its tone should continue to be pleasing and not harsh. Check out the examples below.

∎ **The sense of urgency.** Most TV, radio, and print ads include a sense of urgency so that the viewer, listener, or reader will "act fast" on the offer. In ads for merchandise examples include "Act Today," "This is a limited time offer!," "Sale Ends Wednesday," or "Come in today, when this supply is gone...it's gone forever...don't be left out."

For PCA posters, index card notices, and newspaper ads,

such "hard sell" might be too strong. More realistic examples would include "Help needed now," "Immediate need," "Call today for details," "This apt will go fast." The objective is to get the reader to move quickly to take advantage of the ad while she has the sense of interest and consequent impulse. The "sense of urgency" phrase usually goes between the description of obligation and the contact information.

■ **The contact information.** The most alluring, sexiest ad is useless if information is not provided for contacting the ad's sponsor. The contact info should enable the reader to quickly and easily take advantage of the offer while her interest is peaked.

> The most important part of a newspaper ad or poster is an attractive headline which appeals to a PCA's personal wants & needs -- "Help Wanted" is a dull headline

You have several choices in ways for a PCA to contact you. The best way is the easiest for the PCA -- by phone. If several folks live at the phone number which is listed in the ad, you may wish to also list the first name of the individual who can answer questions. Brief the other people at your phone number about the importance of writing down names and phone numbers of ad respondents who might call in your absence. Even though a phone reply is preferred, some folks choose to protect their privacy by offering a box number address to which PCAs can respond in writing. It is not wise to provide a last name or a street address as contact information to your home, since a weirdo or salesman may decide to visit the for reasons other than for applying for the PCA position.

Newspaper Ads & Newsletter Notices

A classified or display advertisement in a newspaper or organization's newsletter can be very cost effective. By "cost effective," we mean that you should consider 2 factors: the price of the ad and the number of potential PCAs who can be reached by the ad. The ad might at first seem to be expensive, however you might receive several responses. If we divide the price of the ad by the number of people who read it, the "cost per PCA inquiry" is usually very inexpensive.

For example, a newspaper ad that is run for 5 days in a large city might cost $50. If that ad is effectively worded and gets you 25 inquiries, then the "cost per inquiry" is just $2...and the $50 is probably deductible on your personal income taxes as a medically-related expense.

In addition, placing an ad is easier for you than creating, reproducing, and posting notices and posters.

In choosing a newspaper or newsletter, consider at least 2 primary factors:

1) Ask yourself what kind of individual you are seeking as a PCA and therefore which of the area papers that type of individual is likely to read. For example, if you are targetting students at the local college campus, most students will probably read the campus paper. If you want to attract home health aides or nursing assistants who live in the general community and who might want to earn extra money from an extra job, then you might want to advertise in the local community newspaper.

2) If more than one newspaper or newsletter is being read by your target group, compare advertising rates and terms for placing ads. Remember to consider both the price and the size of the readership.

You can use newspaper ads to recruit PCAs in the locale where you now live as well as in an area to which you will soon be moving. You might find it necessary to move to a new part of the same city or even across the country because of changes in school, work, health, or vacation sites. When you are physically dependent upon PCA assistance, sometimes it is essential to recruit help in advance of moving so that the PCA is hired and available for assistance when you first arrive in your new locality.

With a newspaper ad, a PCA can be successfully recruited, interviewed, and hired -- sight unseen -- from even 3,000 miles away! The first step in "long-distance hiring" is to call ahead to the school you will attend, to a contact you have at your new place of work, or to any other contact in the new locale and ask for the name, address, and phone number of the one or two most widely read newspapers on the campus or in that area. The next step is simply to call that paper's classified ad office and explain that you would like details for placing an ad by phone.

Whether you use a local newspaper or one across the country, call the paper or get a recent issue in order to research the details, deadlines, rates, and forms of payment they will accept for placing ads. Ask the particular newspaper about any discount they might offer with certain types or frequency of ads purchased. Also ask about which days of the week have the most and least number of readers -- Thurdays, Fridays, Saturdays, and Sundays are usually the days of heaviest readership for daily papers.

Some people are satisfied with simply dictating the contents of their ad over the phone, telling the clerk which dates the ad should run, and then finding out the price. Other folks prefer to write out their ad and experiment with attractive layouts. Some papers will agree to send a statement to you for your later payment by personal check, while others will require advance payment in person or by giving them a credit card number by phone when the ad is placed.

If you decide to use a newspaper ad, compose your ad after reading the previous section "Some Secrets of Advertising." You will want to experiment with your own ad so it not only conveys your needs but makes working for you sound attractive. Here are some examples of attractive ads for various types of jobs to give you ideas for creating your own ads.

WEEKLY SALARY $5/hr on campus, hours flexible to fit your schedule; female wheelchair student in SIU dorm seeks help in Pierce or Tappan Hall with personal needs; immediate need; write Bx 110 c/o The Campus Times.

EXTRA MONEY $5.50/hr at West Campus dorms this fall; male whchr student will need help at Sleeper or Shelton Hall with living activities; mature M or F apply by 8/15; write Jim, Bx 403, Johnstown, NY 12069.

HOME HEALTH AIDE, earn $5.50 w/flexible hours in Fonda; help senior in her home w/bathing, laundry, cleaning; please apply soon. Betty, 835-8562

FREE FURN APT Boston in classic Back Bay, v-modern w/full kit & 2 bdrms; share in return for live-in help to college male in whchr (2-3 hrs/day); mature M only, need now; call Steve aft 6pm, 553-5354.

CASH TO QUINCY COMMUTER $20 wkly to a Quincy-Boston commuter, your car or mine; C-Zone 9-5 wrkr in wheelchair needs ride wkdays; please call Emery or Gary this week, lv name & # w/sec if not in, 353-3658/3691.

SUMMER $ & MEALS, $6/hr plus meals from 6/1-8/30; vacationing man in whchr needs help in Chattanooga summer home; please write by 4/30; Joseph I., Box 19, Eureka, CA 96941.

Posters and Index Card Notices

A truly inexpensive way to advertise your own PCA job is by putting up posters or index card notices in areas frequented by the type of individual who might be interested in a PCA job. These areas include college campuses, medical facilities, and, less successfully, community bulletin boards found in supermarkets and other general public places. Not only can posted notices be less expensive than newspaper ads, but they can be much faster in getting results.

A true story is told about a college student who, suddenly one morning, needed to immediately replace a live-in PCA who shared his dorm room. As a result of putting up posters in several dorms and cafeterias that morning, a new PCA was actually moved in and on-the-job that same evening!

The objective for posting any notice is to maximize the number of applications which you will receive by increasing the chances that many people will read the notice. The following factors will contribute to accomplishing this objective:

a) Choose posting areas or bulletin boards that have a reputation for being read routinely by many people.

If the building where you wish to post a notice offers only one or two bulletin boards, then you will not have much problem in choosing which boards to use. However, you might be advertising your PCA position on a college campus or in an entire community where a hundred or more boards might be available. In that case you need to decide which locations have the most marketing potential.

> If you are serious about wanting good recruiting results, and you decide to use poster recruiting, then take the time to design & clearly letter a bright-color poster that attracts readers and is easily read from 10' away

You might decide to advertise throughout the entire campus or community, or you might prioritize those bulletin boards that would most likely be read by the type of individual that you would like as a PCA. For example, if your college offers a nursing program and you believe many nursing students are looking for part-time jobs and would make good PCAs, then find a bulletin board likely to be read by these students. This might be in the hallway of the building where nursing classes are held, or in the residence hall where nursing students have rooms.

In addition, choose boards in areas where people stand or sit in order to wait for something -- a hallway area where people wait for elevator cars to arrive, inside the elevator car where people ride, a cafeteria line, or in a lounge or reception area. When folks have to wait and pass time in such an area, they tend to be bored and will read anything they can find...especially notices which are attractive and that apply to their own needs and desires! As another strategy, choose boards which people will directly face as they walk by, sit, or wait in line.

b) Honor restrictions regarding posting notices and posters.

When information is to be posted on a cork bulletin or notice board on a college campus, personnel office, shopping mall, supermarket, or similar area, sometimes there are clearly printed restrictions regarding the type of notice and its size. If the posting area is small, posters are often not allowed and notices must be printed on index cards. There might also be restrictions regarding the type of messages which may be posted, such as "Ride Notices Only," "Housing Notices Only," or "Psychology Department News Only." The sponsor of the bulletin board may even require that all notices be taken to a specific office to receive an approval stamp. If any of these restrictions are in effect where you wish to post notices, it is wise to honor the restrictions or your notice might be soon torn down.

c) Locate your poster or notice card so it can be easily seen.

Your message will be read by more people if it isn't lost within a sea of other notices on a crowded cork board. Bulletin board ethics state that removing the notices of others is OK if those notices have expired. In order to make space for your notice, you may remove other notices which announce events that have already occurred. Additionally, your poster should be mounted without covering someone

Methods for Recruiting PCAs

else's notice. Try to clear sufficient space so that your notice will appear with at least a 1/2" border of bulletin board appearing on all 4 sides of your poster.

d) When mounting posters or index cards, bring a stapler.

Mount your notice securely on the cork boards. Bring a sufficiently loaded stapler and staple your poster with at least one staple in each of the 4 corners.

Do not use tape or thumb tacks to mount your posters. If the next individual wants to mount his notice and hasn't brought a tack or stapler, he will be tempted either to tear down your notice in order to use your thumb tack or to remove your thumb tack, cover your notice with his, and replace the tack through both notices without yours showing.

e) Make your poster colorful, attractive, and easy to read.

Choose paper colors, print colors, headings, and an overall design which will attract readers and make your message easy to read quickly. The next time you pass by a crowded bulletin board, take a moment to see which posters stand out from the others and, in contrast, which ones blend together and are difficult to find. The following features make posters and index card notices more vivid:

■ **Bright-color paper.** Poster cardboard, xerox and mimeograph paper, and index cards all come in a wide variety of bright colors at usually no additional cost over plain white. Choose a color that is bright and yet sufficiently light to show black print.

■ **Wide, dark headings of sufficient size.** If, for example, you have chosen a bright yellow paper, consider a good-sized heading clearly printed with a red marker pen. The heading should be clearly printed (avoid script or fancy calligraphy), and in sufficiently wide and tall letters to be seen from at least 10' away. Avoid printing letters which are the skinny width of pencil or pen. For lettering, use a color of ink which contasts with the light color of your poster paper, for example, avoid using a dark blue marker heading on a blue paper.

■ **Neatly lettered body.** After the large heading, the body of the poster should be neatly lettered. This fine detail of the poster or index card can be typed, preferably in cap letters. The main body should not be handwritten in longhand or handprinted unless the handwriting is exceptionally neat and clear. The message should be either brief or broken up into several, separate phrases, sentences, or paragraphs.

■ **Easily read, overall design.** The poster or card should be neat, pleasing to the eye, and easy to quickly read. A casual reader may be attracted by the colored paper and heading. If she steps up to the poster or card and finds the message difficult to read, she will quit and walk on.

f) Choose wording which will be attractive and appealing to the needs and desires of PCAs. Use words which create a favorable image for the PCA job, and which provide a complete message that is clear, truthful, and descriptive.

Read over the previous section on Advertising Secrets and carefully choose attractive wording for both a heading and the body's main message.

For posters and index card notices, the methods of production, reproduction, and posting should be chosen for four primary considerations:

a) Your degree (and desire) of artistic creativity for the notice's design,
b) Your physical capabilities to design, draw, and letter notices,
c) The number of posters or notices you wish to post, and
d) The time and budget restraints that apply to these tasks.

You should be concerned with producing a clearly written and printed poster which attracts attention and then quickly draws the reader to your employment offer. Of course, feel free to use physical assistance from the PCA whom you now use or a friend for any of the production, reproduction, or posting steps which are beyond your abilities.

> For a few cents each, attractive, colorful, clearly readable posters can be easily printed on bright paper with many photocopy machines

◆Hand-lettered posters on colored stock are effective when just one or two posters are necessary.

◆Hand-typed or word-processed index card notices on colored cards are used where posting restrictions limit the size of notices to be posted on a bulletin board.

◆When a quantity of posters is required, the quick, cost efficient method for producing and reproducing involves using a photocopy machine. The strategy calls for making a master copy of your poster and then photocopying as many copies as needed at the charge of only 5, 10, or 15 cents per poster.

Here are some steps to quickly making a quantity of very effective but inexpensive recruiting posters:

1) When a quantity of posters is required, start by making a clear master which will be photocopied. Use white paper of the same size which is accepted by the photocopy machine, usually the standard 8 1/2" x 11". A higher quality paper of 18 or 20-pound weight and with a 25% rag content will "soak up" your typewriter or computer-printer ink and give you a sharp copy. Avoid using coated or erasable paper for the master copy. Use a typewriter, word processor, or graphics computer program which produces a clearly printed copy.

2) Either of 2 kinds of a master can be made: a complete poster which includes all of the poster's content, or a partial poster in which a blank space is left for any part of the poster which will be later hand-lettered on each copy. In the latter case, a larger, bright-color marker heading or border can be hand-lettered on each poster which has been produced by the photocopy machine; this helps draw attention of readers.

3) Design and type out the master similar to the example shown below. Contact information tear-tabs should border one of the edges to make it easy for PCA respondents to tear off your phone number and call you later.

4) When the master is complete, photocopy the posters. Use colored paper stock for the copies when possible; many copy services offer color stock at no extra charge. Ask to see the first copy before others are printed to be sure the print is sufficiently dark.

5) For each resulting poster copy, add any desired hand-lettered parts in bright colored marker. Use scissors to cut slits between each of the contact information tear-tabs. These tabs will make it easy for someone who is interested in your PCA job to rip off a tab and call you later. The unfortunate alternatives include a prospect taking your entire poster just for its phone number, or inaccurately copying your phone number.

6) Put up the posters with a stapler as discussed in the previous section.

Here are examples of effective posters and bulletin board notices:

Poster example:

FREE FURNISHED APT

*Boston, in classic Coolidge Corner, within qtr block of Beacon trolley stop
*Very modern, full kitchen, 8th floor, north & west balcony views
*Share in return for live-in help to working, college-age male of wheelchair mobility (2-3 hrs/day)
*Mature males only, non-smoking, no drugs
*No experience necessary -- Needed right away!!!

Please call Earl after 6pm for details, 277-7033

| Earl aft 6pm 277-7033 | Earl aft 6pm 277-7033 | Earl aft 6pm 277-7033 | Earl aft 6pm 277-7033 | Earl aft 6pm 277-7033 | Earl aft 6pm 277-7033 | Earl aft 6pm 277-7033 |

(cut a vertical slit between tear-tabs)

Index card notice example:

(entire message typed onto bright-colored index card)

$80 EXTRA EACH MONTH for JUST 4 1/2 HRS EACH WEEK !

A 38-year old female of wheelchair mobility needs physical assistance with morning dressing and grooming on 3 mornings each week (M-W-F, 7-8:30am).
My husband (able-bodied) and I live in Seattle just 5 minutes from downtown. He needs a rest from assisting me and I would like to hire an aide who is punctual and dependable.
We need help now.
Call 762-8941 (9-5) or 853-3219 (after 6pm) for details, ask for Patricia; please leave message on machine if no answer.

Describing the PCA Job by Word-of-Mouth or by Phone.

It is important to be able to verbally express the details of your need for PCA help in a concise manner during both informal conversations and over the phone.

In examining various methods for recruiting, a very effective means is by your everyday word-of-mouth conversations with friends, fellow students, co-workers, neighbors, and current PCAs. When you are actively recruiting, ask these folks whether they would be interested in considering helping you or whether they know of anyone who would. Some very responsible people whom you might not believe are interested might surprise you with their personal interest or contacts.

The ability to represent the PCA position by phone is often useful for either of 2 situations:

a) For making your own inquiries, when you are calling a home health aide agency, a previous PCA contact, or someone whom you heard might be interested in the job, or

b) For replying to individuals who are responding to your newspaper ad, poster, or bulletin board notice.

If you are like most of us, and you are not instantly "verbally organized on-demand," like a rapid-fire radio DJ, you will find it very helpful to organize and prepare a bit of information before you make or receive that first phone call. The preparation will take just a few minutes and will result in your making a well-organized, first impression to others, while being a lot less nervous and much more confident.

We suggest that you prepare in advance along the following guidelines:

1) Examine your job description and write out some very brief notes which cover the following:

    a) Your physical condition and age,
    b) Your living situation,
    c) The broad categories (but not fine, step-by-step details)

Methods for Recruiting PCAs

of the specific duties which the PCA will be performing,
d) The days of the week and overall schedule of hours for the needed help, and
e) The monetary salary you are offering.

2) Telephone information should be neither detailed nor lengthy unless you are answering detailed questions. You should edit your notes so the initial verbal presentation takes no more than about a minute. If the PCA prospect or home health agency wants more detailed information, by all means feel free to expand the details. However, most sources will need initially just an outline of you and your needs. Think of them as initially asking you "What time is it?" In response, give them the time; don't tell them how to build a watch!

Here are examples of an appropriate amount of initial detail:

"I'm a quadriplegic who is 38 years old and who uses a motorized wheelchair because of a diving injury several years ago. I'm very active each day and I need assistance on Monday, Wednesday, and Friday mornings from 7-8:30. The help which I need is for dressing, transferring from bed to wheelchair, and cooking a simple breakfast. Does this sound like the type of work in which you are interested?".

or

"My mother is 82 years old and had a stroke 2 years ago. She lives with me, but cannot take care of all her needs. I need someone to help my mother get bathed and dressed each weekday morning. I'm paying $5.50 an hour. Does this sound like the type of work in which you are interested?"

> Practice to yourself the words you will use to briefly & concisely express your PCA job to prospects who call you

3) Before expressing your needs to someone else, while you are by yourself and mistakes don't matter, practice the content and delivery of your brief presentation. You should use an easy-going, comfortable pace with clear articulation. Don't mumble and don't race through the details.

4) Be prepared to supply further details as requested or as otherwise appropriate.

Further detail and procedural steps in determining whether a PCA prospect is interested in the job, and if so what to do next, are provided in the chapter "Interviewing, Screening, and Hiring Prospective PCAs."

Interviewing, Screening, & Hiring Prospective PCAs   279

26. Interviewing, Screening, & Hiring Prospective PCAs

Objectives for Interviewing & Screening.

The objective of recruiting is to attract responsible and qualified people to apply for your PCA position. The objective of interviewing and screening is to determine which applicants (if any) sufficiently meet your standards, and therefore to determine which applicants merit hiring. In addition, it is in your best interest for the PCA applicant to learn all the essential information about you and the job duties, and therefore she can knowledgeably decide whether she is able and willing to perform the job duties. During the face-to-face interview, you should NOT try to hide any important but less pleasant details about the job in order to make the job seem more attractive.

> A good interview enables you to learn about the applicant, and the applicant to learn about you & the job

Here are 3 primary goals which you can achieve from this chapter:

1) To know which personal traits in applicants to avoid and which are favorable,

2) To know how to observe and screen applicants for these traits during either face-to-face interviews or the phone interviews required for hiring PCAs who already live in a new locale to which you are moving, and

3) To know the basic step-by-step procedure for setting up an interview, observing personal traits of applicants, checking references, ranking preferences of applicants after the interviews, and hiring some applicants while rejecting others.

Applicant Traits to Favor and Avoid.

A quite comprehensive list of favorable and unfavorable traits in PCAs is shown in a previous chapter "Job

Expectations." In that chapter, there are two listings of favorable traits...one for you as the employer and one for the PCA who assists you. Next to each favorable trait is the contrasting, negative consequence of not having or providing that trait.

In preparing yourself for interviewing, screening, and hiring, we suggest that you review that previous chapter. Additionally, here is a recap of the primary traits that a good PCA has and which you should look for during interviews.

■ **An understanding of the nature & responsibility of the work.** A PCA prospect must have an understanding of the nature and responsibility of providing you with the very personal assistance upon which you are so dependent. This understanding can come from previous PCA experience or from your careful explanation of the seriousness of the work involved.

■ **Dependability.** You should be able to rely and depend upon the PCA coming to work on the schedule for which you have both agreed. "No shows" are both inexcusable and unethical to someone who is physically and medically dependent upon assistance as you are. If the PCA prospect does not appear at all for his interview, then he is not worth your effort to re-establish contact; you will not want to employ him.

■ **Punctuality.** In addition to being dependable, it is important that a PCA values arriving at (or a bit before) the starting time for each work session, or calls in advance to notify you of his inability to do so. During interviews, observe whether each prospect is punctual in arriving for their scheduled interview appointment. If not, the prospect might be similarly lax in not arriving for routine work on time.

■ **A clean and reasonably neat appearance.** A PCA should be clean and neat in not appearing with dirty clothing, greasy or otherwise "grubby" hair, foul body odor, unsanitary "mannerisms," or dirty and greasy hands, fingernails, or skin. Why? First, it will not be pleasant to work closely with him. Second, if he does not care about keeping his own body and clothes clean, he will not care very much about helping you stay clean. During the interview, check out the appearance of each prospect.

■ **A clear, logical, and rational head.** We are not addressing the IQ-level of intelligence of each prospect, but instead whether "he has his own act together" sufficiently well to then be able to help you with your physical needs. Some people have an inherent inability to think logically and reasonably remember work details and schedules. Other folks have those abilities, but are too strung out on alcohol, prescription medications, or street drugs to use those abilities. The negative consequences of hiring either type of PCA are obvious to your need for a clear thinker. During the interview, listen carefully to the PCA's answers to your questions...answers which should be logical and clearly answer the specific questions asked. Avoid someone who rambles on and on without thinking.

■ **No evidence of substance abuse.** To further confirm the need for a clear thinker, be on the lookout for abuse of alcohol, prescription medications, and street drugs. For an applicant to come to a job interview while even slightly "under the influence" will be a pretty reliable indication that the applicant has a substance dependency which will show up more seriously during routine work. If there is ANY such evidence during the job interview, do NOT hire the prospect...no matter how charming her personality or how sorrowful her "hard times" sob story.

■ **A pleasant personality.** No one has an ideal personality, but a good PCA should have a sufficiently favorable personality so that you can tolerate working with her. During the interview, watch out for extremes during your conversations. Extremes include either the sugary, syrupy, "isn't life wonderful" do-good prospect, or the sarcastic, harsh, intimidating, "mad at the world" tough prospect. Be attracted to the comfortable personality of someone who is confident-and-yet-humble while showing you her true self.

■ **A good listener who respects you and your methods.** A good PCA will listen to information which you convey to her in a clear, direct, assertive manner (see the previous chapter "Passive, Aggressive, Assertive..."). An undesirable PCA is not interested in your opinion, concerns, or preferred methods and schedule for your needs. During the interview, observe whether each prospect is sincerely interested in you and your opinions, or whether she couldn't care less and merely will want her paycheck. You have a good brain and the ability to know and express your needs. If you are "able-minded," you should be the best authority on the types of assistance which you require as well as the safest and most efficient methods for providing that assistance. See whether each prospect recognizes those facts, or will tend to insist on "caring for you" and performing tasks her way.

■ **Appropriate reasons for wanting the job.** Appropriate reasons include needing the cash or noncash salary, a desire for friendship, and a reasonable desire to provide you with the assistance which you need. Besides receiving a monetary salary, the PCA should be the kind of individual who likes the satisfaction and personal reward which come from doing a job well and taking pride in detail. Inappropriate reasons include wanting to cure your ailment, to be your psychological counselor, to single-handedly provide all of your assistance for a lifetime, to obtain sexual favors (inappropriate if that desire is not mutual), to use freely or steal your medications, possessions, food, or friends, or to verbally or physically control or abuse you. During the interview, ask clearly and directly "Why do you want this job?," and see if you get a clear, straightforward, and appropriate answer.

■ **A sense of respect and confidentiality for you and your personal information.** A good PCA should never discuss with others the details of your personal needs, values, relations with others, possessions, or similar factors which comprise "gossip." During the interview, observe whether any of your prospects relate to you any gossip-type details about other people whom they have assisted. If so, you can assume that they will be similarly free in spreading details of your own lifestyle...if you hire them.

Interview Observation Skills from Sherlock Holmes.

The legendary, literary detective Sherlock Holmes has been noted for his keen ability to observe personal traits, mannerisms, and preferences of others, and consequently to predict their behavior for the future. Wouldn't it be great to hire Mr. Holmes to sit in with you on PCA interviews, quietly observe, and later advise you about which applicants to hire and which to avoid?

Well, we have consulted some notes from Mr. Holmes as well as people who have conducted many kinds of face-to-face interviews. Here are some very valuable strategies for learning a wealth of information about the PCA applicant who will be sitting in front of you.

> Observe personal traits & listen to how something is said in addition to what is said

There are 7 primary factors which will increase your ability to learn everything possible from each applicant. These should be kept in mind while following the detailed interview procedure which is listed later in this chapter.

1) Make the applicant feel comfortable so she will be candid in her answers,

2) Observe her nonverbal personal traits and behavior,

3) Listen to what she says as well as how she says it,

4) Ask specific questions, watch her reactions, and listen to her answers,

5) Invite the applicant to ask her own questions, and observe her reaction and level of interest,

6) Check employment and character references,

7) Rely on your "6th sense"; trust your gut reaction and intuition.

1) Make each applicant feel comfortable during the interview. When you read through the upcoming interview procedure, there will be suggestions that you should allow the applicant to sit comfortably, be friendly toward the applicant, and that you begin the interview with "ice breaker" questions and conversation. These suggestions contribute to your image as a nice individual for whom the candidate might work, and equally important, they make the applicant comfortable so that her answers to your questions will be more open and revealing. One of your interview goals is to see the real applicant as they routinely behave, and not a nervous individual who guards their answers and hides their true personality traits with "ideal behavior."

2) Observe her nonverbal personal traits and behavior. If you were Sherlock Holmes, you would be interested in what an applicant's visible habits tell you as well as in her verbal answers to questions.

    a) Punctuality -- did she arrive for the interview appointment on time (or a bit before), or did she arrive late and full of excuses,

    b) Appearance -- was she reasonably neat and clean, or greasy and dirty,

    c) Mannerisms -- was she reasonably cool, collected, logical, and organized, or was she extremely nervous, erratic in gestures, and perhaps "spaced out,"

    d) Eye contact -- did she look at you and into your eyes with a pleasant and confident face as she spoke, or did she avoid looking at you as much as possible?

3) Listen to what she says as well as how she says it.

    a) Clarity of voice -- did she speak with reasonable clarity so that you could easily hear and communicate with her, or did she mumble so low that she couldn't be heard and possibly didn't care or want to be heard,

    b) Clarity of answers -- were her answers to your questions logical and reasonably organized on the topic of your questions, or did she ramble in an unorganized way on information which didn't answer your questions,

    c) Tone of voice -- was her speaking tone pleasant and reasonably respectful of you as an intelligent individual and potential employer, or did her tone convey disgust, arrogance, and a clear lack of reasonable respect for you,

d) Attitude toward work and helping you -- did her combination of tone and clarity of answers tell you that she was really interested in the work and willing to help you, or did she seem uninterested and uncommitted to wanting the job?

4) Ask questions, watch reactions, and listen to answers. The upcoming interview procedure will suggest certain questions for you to ask, and certainly you will have your own to add. Sherlock Holmes fans have noticed that the companion to Mr. Holmes, Dr. Watson, usually just listens to the actual content of what someone says. Holmes additionally concentrates on someone's visible reaction to questions as they are posed. Both the content and personal reaction are often useful in determining how someone truly feels about a topic which he is discussing.

5) Invite the applicant to ask her own questions and observe her reaction and level of interest. In most good interviews, there is time provided for the applicant to ask his own questions. These questions can provide him with the opportunity to acquire the information which he needs to decide whether he wants the job. Additionally, his visible reaction and degree of enthusiasm to this opportunity can often reveal his degree of interest in the job.

6) Check employment and character references. There will be a specific part of the upcoming interview procedure which addresses ways to check references of an applicant. Checking references gives you very important information about each applicant.

7) Rely on your "6th sense"; trust your gut reaction and intuition. Perhaps the most important indicator of an interview is "how you feel" about each applicant. Regardless of someone's very impressive and visible surface, ask your intuition whether you are comfortable with each candidate and believe that you can trust them to have been truly representative of themselves.

A very successful businessman was recently asked in a magazine interview for a single, important piece of advice to offer to others in business. His reply: "Never hire or keep an employee whom you don't like...if you don't like him, it's probably because you don't believe you can trust him. Your instincts are probably valid; sooner or later he'll screw you."

Step-by-Step Procedure.

To this point, we have discussed the objectives for interviewing and screening, which applicant traits to favor and avoid, and some tips from Sherlock Holmes on how to observe as much as possible from the applicant who sits in front of you during an interview.

Now, let's get on with the actual interview!

The actual procedure for interviewing, screening, and hiring will vary with each employment situation. There is no single formula for conducting an interview. The steps listed below should be viewed as one way of proceeding, and therefore merely as a guideline for interviewing which you might conduct.

Compare the interviewing procedure to sketching or painting a work of art. The list of steps which follow can be viewed as one way to paint a picture, so that you can get a "feel" for one approach to painting. After you are familiar with this particular procedure, set it aside and develop a personal style with which you are comfortable and that works for you and your specific employment objectives and situation.

> There is no single "best" procedure for conducting interviews; this one will give you format ideas for developing your own style

1) You receive replies to your recruiting. A prospect calls or writes you, mentions seeing your job notice, and expresses interest in learning more about the PCA job offering.

You thank her for calling and give her a brief (one minute maximum) introduction to the job, with points such as these:

   a) Your medical condition and type of disability

b) The categories (but not details) of duties for which you need physical assistance, and the schedule of days and times when that assistance is needed

c) Your need for someone who is dependable and punctual

d) The amount of cash or noncash salary you are offering

Examples of informative introductions to PCA jobs include:

"I'm a quadriplegic who is 38 years old and who uses a motorized wheelchair because of a diving injury several years ago. I'm very active each day and I need assistance on Monday, Wednesday, and Friday mornings from 7-8:30. The help which I need is for dressing, transferring from bed to wheelchair, and cooking a simple breakfast. Does this sound like the type of work in which you are interested?".

or

"My mother is 82 years old and had a stroke 2 years ago. She lives with me, but cannot take care of all her needs. I need someone to help my mother get bathed and dressed each weekday morning. I'm paying $5.50 an hour. Does this sound like the type of work in which you are interested?"

2) You ask if this is a position in which she might be interested and would like more information. Save yourself from providing 5 minutes of further details to someone who has already decided that your job isn't what he, personally, wants. This is no time to become a pushy, rapid-talk salesman who fears that if the customer gets a chance to speak, he will turn down the sale!

At this point, a number of callers might tell you that they are not interested in the personal type of work, schedule, or possibly the level or type of salary. Don't try to talk him out of his decision; respect the caller for being straightforward even though you might be disappointed. You should expect to screen out some people at this phone inquiry time. Don't become discouraged. If the caller is not interested, you thank him for calling.

3) If the caller is interested, you ask some introductory questions. The answers which you receive will determine whether you are interested in offering him a chance to meet (interview) with you. If possible, start taking written notes about his answers to the following types of questions which you ask on the phone:

a) Ask whether he has done this kind of work before

- If so, ask what kind of work he performed, where, when, and for how long,

- If not, explain that experience is not essential because you will teach the PCA whom you hire about your specific needs, however what is essential is that someone without experience in this work realizes the personal nature of the work and that he must be very dependable and reliable. Next ask what other kind of work he has done.

b) Ask in which town, city, or section of your city he lives, whether he has a car, and if not how he would intend to arrive to your home on a routine and punctual basis.

c) Ask whether he smokes, if this is a concern to you, and if he does smoke whether he will mind not smoking while he is in your college dorm room, apartment, or house.

d) If there is physical lifting involved in your routine, explain the details and ask whether he is physically capable of assisting you.

4) If all has gone well to this point, you have 2 choices:

a) To state that you are taking notes about those who respond over the next few days, and that you will be calling back a couple of those people during this week. You get the caller's phone number and thank him for calling. Tell them that you might be calling him in about a week (or whatever an appropriate amount of time might be).

This choice is appropriate when either you actually are taking notes about respondents because you expect several applicant calls and you intend to call back the top couple of applicants, or the caller is someone whom you obviously do not want to consider hiring because of their inappropriate attitude, work experience, or a negative or uneasy feeling which you have about them.

b) Or, to ask whether he would like to meet with you right away to discuss in more detail the duties, schedule, and salary.

This choice is appropriate when you do not believe that you will be receiving numerous applications and the present caller has impressed you.

> Expect that between 1/4 and 3/4 of all prospects who enthusiastically make interview appointments with you will be "no shows" This is their problem and not yours. Don't become personally offended or discouraged

5) Arrange for an interview.

Interviews are important to enable you to meet each serious applicant, make personal observations, ask in-depth questions about the applicant, and fully explain the duties. An interview also allows the applicant to decide whether he wants the job which you might offer him.

The PCA interview is usually a face-to-face meeting at your residence. However, if you are moving to a distant locale, and wish to interview a PCA who lives in that new area, you can easily conduct an interview by phone. If the interview is conducted by phone, it can be accomplished during the initial call in which the PCA inquires about your job or the interview can be scheduled for a later call.

Since most interviews are accomplished with face-to-face meetings, the next procedural steps will refer to meeting-type interviews. If you are interviewing "long distance" by phone, simply adapt the details of meeting-type interviews to what can be done by phone.

Whether you are conducting an interview during the applicant's initial call of inquiry. or you selectively call back two or three applicants, the procedure is the same. You start by asking whether she would like to meet with you to discuss in more detail the duties, schedule, salary, and other details.

You will probably receive one of 3 replies:

    a) If she clearly states that she does not wish to meet with you, simply thank her for calling.

    b) If she seems uneasy and unwilling to make a yes/no decision regarding meeting with you, you might advise her that she probably needs more time to think about the position, and that she should feel free to call you back if she wishes. Thank her for calling, but realize that you will probably not hear again from her.

    c) If she does wish to meet with you, propose a day and specific time which is convenient to you, and be ready to compromise to a reasonable degree if that date is not convenient to her. Ask for her full name, address, and phone number before giving her yours and the directions for meeting with you. Just before hanging up, restate the day and time of your meeting, tell her that you will be waiting for her at that time and if she cannot come, decides not to come, or knows that she will be late, that you ask that she calls you in as much advance as possible.

6) PCA interview "no shows" are common. The objective for the interview appointment is both to interview those who might make good PCAs and to weed out those who are irresponsible and not serious about the job. You can expect that between 1/4 and 3/4 of all prospects who make such appointments, and have sworn to you and the Godfather that they desperately want the job, will neither call nor show up for the appointment. Expect this inconsideration to occur and do not take it personally.

Do not waste your time in trying to call back a "no show" to reprimand her and try to arrange a 2nd interview. She has shown you that she is irresponsible and too passive to verbally state that she has decided not to interview. Cross these prospects off your list and recruite some new ones.

7) Greet the interview applicant. To those who do come for their appointment on time (or nearly so), be cordial, friendly, and make them comfortable. Your objective is to find a good employee and not to rudely "interrogate" someone in order to "show them who is boss." Greet them with a smile, invite them to be comfortable, and show them a place to sit which you have pre-planned. Remember that you probably need them more than they need you, so assume that they will be an excellent PCA (unless they clearly show you otherwise), and impress them with what a reasonably friendly individual you would be for whom to work. Treat them as a highly valued employee before you even get acquainted. Some other communication tips include:

   a) Speak clearly and at a moderate (not rushed) pace

   b) Smile, keep your chin up, and make good eye contact

   c) Frequently ask whether the applicant has any questions, and be a good listener when questions are raised

   d) Be careful during the discussions not to address the applicant as if she may assume that she has been hired. Use phrases such as "if you took this job" or "if you are the individual whom I hire," instead of "you will find this job easy to learn" or "when you arrive each morning to help me..." Use phrases in the conditional tense, instead of implying that the applicant can assume that she will be or has been hired.

   If the applicant hears that she seems to have been already hired, you might lose control of the interview. Additionally, if she believes she has been hired and then is not actually hired, she might end up both confused and mad.

8) Points to ask & discuss with each candidate. As she sits down and becomes comfortable, thank her for coming and ask a few friendly "ice breaker" questions ("How's the weather?," "Did you have trouble finding my place?," "That's a neat jacket...did you get it around here?").

After she loosens up and begins to smile, state that you would like to provide her with information on the following topics, however you will welcome questions at anytime:

a) Introduce yourself

b) Ask a few details about the applicant

c) Outline to the PCA applicant the qualities which you seek in a PCA

d) Describe the duties and schedule with which you need physical help, while you provide her with your written job description (or at least your written list and schedule of needs). It might also help the applicant to visualize the routine if you physically walk the her through the rooms where she will be assisting you and

e) Discuss the salary

a) Introduce yourself.

Be appropriately brief and spare them from hearing more detail than they need or want to hear. Approximately 1 or 2 minutes should do it.

▪ Your age (if you don't mind)
▪ Your occupation, student status, or other routine type of daily activity
▪ A brief description of your disabiity, its cause, date of onset
▪ Your sensory and motor (feeling and muscular) abilities & inabilities

b) Ask a few details about the applicant

There are 3 objectives here which will enable later comparing candidates and ranking them according to your hiring preferences:

1) To promote a friendly discussion with the applicant so that she will be comfortable with you and be more candid when answering questions,

2) To acquire specific factual information to determine the individual's qualifications for the PCA job, and

3) To enable listening to and observing non-factual information about the applicant to determine the applicant's attitude toward you and the job.

Choose topics which are appropriate for each applicant. Some affirmative-action and equal-opportunity purists will argue that some of the topics below are not geared toward objectively determining one's ability to perform a job description. That might be true for a bureaucratic office job. However, let's remember the personal, close working nature of PCA work and the very negative emotional effects to you of requesting assistance from a PCA who has a negative attitude or unfavorable personality.

> Make interview candidates comfortable and they will "open up" and show you more about their true selves

The topics below are suggestions for determining an applicant's qualifications to perform the job, ability to arrive at work reliably and punctually, and to learn about the applicant's ability to personally interact smoothly with the employer whom they will be assisting. Topic suggestions include asking about

■ The geographical area where they were raised and their personal background: "Tell me a little about yourself, Susan, did you grow up around here?," "What do you like to do in your spare time?"
■ Schooling, education, professional training: "What is your educational background?," "Where did you go to school?"
■ Work history: "What kind of work have you done in the past?," "Where did you work?," "For how long?," "What did you like and not like about each job?"
■ Transportation: "How far away from here do you live?," "Do you have a car?," if not, "How would you be getting to this job on a regular schedule?"
■ Attraction to this job: "Why do you want this job?"

■ Personality: "What kinds of things get you mad?," "What do you do when you get mad?"
■ The future: "What do you see yourself doing 3 or 4 years from now?"

c) Outline to the applicant the qualities and other factors which you seek in a PCA.

Add to these items any other factors which are important to you

■ To be dependable and reliable. Tell the applicant that you are physically dependent on receiving assistance every day (or whatever frequency applies to your situation). Let him know the types of negative consequences which occur if a PCA fails to arrive with either no advance notice or too little advance notice to enable you to find a PCA replacement. Give personal experiences or examples.

Possible summary statement: "A PCA must be dependable and reliable because of my physical dependence on routine help. If circumstances, weather, or sickness will prevent a PCA from arriving as scheduled, then I ask that they call me as much in advance as possible."

■ To be reasonably punctual. Explain to the applicant that at least 2 negative things happen when a PCA is not reasonably punctual in arriving each time. First, you worry that she is not at all coming and that you will not receive the physical assistance upon which you are dependent. Second, that your day's schedule will either start late or be delayed by the amount of time by which the PCA is late. Give personal experiences or examples.

Possible summary statement: "Once more, if circumstances, weather, or sickness will prevent a PCA from arriving within 10 minutes of the scheduled arrival, then I ask that she calls me as much in advance as possible."

■ To be confidential. The applicant will learn many personal facts about you and your assets, possessions, family, and personal concerns. These facts should never leave your living area. Give personal experiences and examples.

Possible summary statement: "If you were to take this job, I would ask that you not discuss outside any topics which are personal to me and that you be discrete about any nonpersonal topics."

■ To be open in discussing work-related concerns. Tell the applicant that you work very closely with the PCAs who assist you and that maintaining a close working relationship is very important. It is essential that the PCA feel free to initiate discussions about concerns, problems, or complaints related to working with you, and that you can feel free to do the same. When problems are raised by PCAs, your reaction is not to become insulted or mad, but instead to want to work with the PCA in resolving the issue in order to improve the working relationship. Give personal experiences and examples.

Possible summary statement: "If you were to take this job, our good relationship would depend on openness from both of us. The biggest danger is to keep problems a secret and let them smolder over time until they explode and the working relationship is lost."

■ To provide you an advance notice of resigning. Explain to the PCA prospect that recruiting responsible help is not easy and requires time. Since you are physically dependent on assistance, you cannot go without it and the supply of help cannot be interrupted. Give personal experiences and examples. Specify your need for a 2, 3, 4, or whatever-weeks advance notice.

Possible summary statement: "Unless a PCA suddenly finds that health or extreme personal crisis causes her to resign on short notice, I would ask that she be fair with me and give me at least a 3 week advance notice of an intention to resign."

d) Describe the duties and schedule with which you need physical help while touring the area of your home where the help will be provided.

With help from your job description, give the PCA applicant a run-through of the duties with the schedule for each. Providing the prospect with her own copy of the job description may be helpful. She can read along with you now, and if she is a serious candidate you can suggest that she reads it again at home and asks any questions which occur.

It may help the PCA if this "tour of duties" is presented within the actual bedroom, bathroom, or other area in which the work will be performed. Cite the list of duties in a logical and chronological order, speak at a moderate and not rushed rate, and ask often if the applicant has any questions.

e) Discuss the salary.

Explain the details of the cash or noncash salary which you are paying. Immediately follow this salary figure with the amount and date of any merit increases which the hired PCA will receive. Address the frequency and standard payday with which checks will be available. Also identify and explain any withholdings which you will or will not be deducting from paychecks.

9) Ask again whether the applicant has any other questions, and take the time to answer the questions thoroughly.

This is NOT a time to hide any unpleasant details in an attempt to make the job seem more attractive.

Ask whether they are still interested in the job. If not, collect their copy of the job description, thank them for coming and walk them to the door. If they are still interested, go to step #10.

10) Get reference contacts from each serious candidate. If you are interested in further considering the applicant, and you do not know the applicant personally, ask the applicant to supply you with at least 2 references from previous employers (not to include friends or relatives). The purpose for the references is to enable you to obtain evaluations of the applicant's character as well as her previous work from other employers.

For each reference, the applicant should supply you with the following information:

a) Name of the reference

This can be the name of an individual who employed the applicant in a private home, or the name and title of a previous supervisor in an agency or institution.

b) Address and phone number (if they can remember the number)

c) Approximate dates of employment with each reference

d) The applicant's job title and job responsibilities under this reference

e) The applicant's opinion as to why she left this previous job

> When you describe the job duties, do not hide the more unpleasant tasks with a fear of scaring away a candidate from wanting the job

11) End the interview in a friendly manner. At this point, state that you are meeting with some other applicants during the next few hours or days, and that after you have made a hiring decision you will be calling each applicant with whom you have met. Thank the party for meeting with you and tell them that you will be calling them within a week (or whatever an appropriate amount of time might be). This choice is appropriate when:

▶You are satisfied with the applicant in front of you, but need a few hours or days to check references and make a decision,

▶You actually are meeting with other applicants, or

▶The applicant with whom you are now meeting is someone whom you obviously do not want to consider hiring because of their inappropriate attitude, work experience, or a negative or uneasy feeling which you have about them. In this situation, you plan to call back the applicant quite soon and reject their application.

12) Check the references. As soon as possible, you should begin checking the references which have been offered to you. Call each reference and:

a) State your name, the fact that you are considering the hire of (state applicant's name) for a job as a home health aide to you, that he has offered this individual you have called as an employment reference, and ask whether you may ask the reference a few brief questions.

b) If so, ask the approximate dates of the applicant's employment with the reference, what position the applicant held, and for what types of duties he was responsible.

c) Ask the reference whether the applicant's work was satisfactory and whether the reference would rehire the applicant.

d) Ask why the applicant left the employment of the reference.

e) Briefly explain that you are considering the hire of the applicant for a home health aide position, that you have a disability, that the applicant would be assisting you with very personal needs, and that the individual assisting you must be reliable, punctual, and confidential with personal information. Ask the reference whether they would have any reservations in hiring the applicant for this type of work.

f) Thank the reference for her help.

13) Call the other references for each applicant whom you are considering, since you will want more than one, unrelated opinion on each applicant.

If you can, take brief notes either during or right after each reference conversation. It is too easy to forget or mix-up details in your head if no written notes are made.

14) Check the information which you receive from the references for at least 2 factors:

   a) Are there any serious discrepancies between facts from the applicant and those from the references? Discrepancies are serious if they show that the applicant was lying to you in an attempt to hide a poor performance record, bad habits, or other undesirable events or traits. They are not serious if discrepancies in small details or exact dates can be excused by an applicant's reasonable lapse of memory.

   b) Are there any significant reasons voiced by the references for advising you not to hire the applicant? Decide whether any of those negative reasons or negative past performance actually applies to the type of work which the applicant will be performing for you.

15) Rank your preferences. After your reference check calls are complete, it is time to compile all of the available information about each applicant whom you are considering (information from the interview, references, and possibly other sources) and put each applicant into one of 3 categories:

   a) Reject -- this applicant is undesirable for PCA work with me at anytime,

   b) Backup file -- this applicant is qualified and desirable for hire, however there is a more desirable applicant at this time, or

   c) Offer employment -- this applicant is the most desirable and qualified and will be the first to be offered the job

16) Update your backup file. For applicants of the "backup file" and "offer employment" categories above, write out some basic notes on each of these folks while you still remember the details of your encounter with them. These favorable applicants can be very important to you, because the people who are desirable but not hired for the current PCA opening are the first people whom you might call:

a) If your first choice, new employee decides not to take the job or proves to be so unsatisfactory in performing duties that you must fire and replace him in the first few days,

b) If your new employee is satisfactory, but temporarily unable to work at any time, due to factors such as sickness or vacation, and you must quickly find a temporary fill-in replacement, and

c) When your new employee eventually decides to resign -- as all employees eventually do -- and you must find another new employee

As outlined in the previous chapter "Sources for Recruiting PCAs," these favorable PCA applicants should be your first contacts the next time that you must recruit either temporary fill-in or more permanent help.

We suggest that you maintain a "backup file" of notes written either on index cards, one card per previous applicant, or on the appropriate word-processing or file/database software of a computer.

Each index card, or computer file, should bear the following information about a favorable PCA applicant:

a) The date of your contact with the applicant,

b) The type of contact (phone, home interview, or other),

c) Whatever biographical information you obtained: name, address, phone number, work experience and duration, whether has car, etc.,

d) Whether applicant is willing to perform temporary fill-in work for you,

e) The salary figure quoted to the applicant, and

f) Your private remarks about your favorable or unfavorable observations and impressions about the applicant.

17) Offer employment (hiring). As soon as your decisions are made, and all of the applicants have been placed into one of the 3 categories of "reject," "backup file," or "offer employment," it is time to call your favorite candidate and offer the job.

> Take the time to write or computer-log a backup file of desirable-but-unused applicants; recruiting future PCAs will be much easier & quicker

The entire process of checking references, making your decisions, and offering the job to the top applicant should be accomplished as quickly as is practical. The reason is that each applicant is probably actively searching for work. If you allow even a whole week or 10 days to pass between interviews and offering employment, then you might find that your top candidate has accepted another job elsewhere.

The job offer should be communicated in a direct, clear, assertive manner, so that the applicant clearly realizes that the offer is being made. "Good morning, Peggy, this is Bill Reardon. If you are still interested in the PCA job, I am calling to offer it to you."

If your favorite candidate accepts your offer, the two of you should agree on a starting date for the immediate future. You should state to the new employee that if she finds that she will be arriving late on the starting date, will be unable at all to come, or decides that she no longer wants the job, she should call you in as much advance as possible. Tell the new employee that you are looking forward to working with her, and end your conversation by repeating the starting date and meeting time when the two of you will start work together.

If your favorite candidate rejects your offer, thank her and call your next favorite candidate from the backup file.

You should successfully hire a PCA before following the next step of making rejection calls. After all, if your top 1 or 2 candidates decide not to take your job, you may decide to dip into your "backup file" of candidates right away.

18) Call to reject other applicants whom you interviewed or to whom you promised a decision. There may be other applicants, besides the one who has accepted the job, whom you interviewed and you believe you should inform of your hiring decision.

For some who are totally undesirable, rejection should be made soon after the interview is concluded. These are the applicants whom you have decided not to employ at anytime. The time-proven phrase which can be used is "I regret that I am unable to hire you at this time." The message is clear and you do not need to give the candidates specific reasons for having rejected them with which they can argue.

For the other, desirables of your backup file, the message is that you have hired someone else, however you would like to keep these candidates in your file for future needs. Ask for their OK to be called when you need backup help in the future, so they will not be totally surprised if you do call them.

You should not be too hasty in making these calls to backups. The key strategy is first to be sure that your newly hired PCA will actually show up for work and will work beyond the first few days. In some circles there is a very slim chance that anything will go wrong with the new PCA; in other circles of especially college students and nursing students, the chance for failure in the first few days can be as high as 50%.

The folks in your backup file are the first ones to call when a replacement is necessary. It would be awkward, and a bit embarrassing, to turn down someone and then to call them 3 days later with a job offer.

You have nothing to gain, and perhaps something to lose, in turning down a "backup file" applicant prematurely. Wait before making these calls to determine whether the new PCA -- your first choice -- shows up for work the first day and then performs satisfactory work for the first 3 or 4 days.

If all goes well, then call back these "backup file" applicants. Be friendly and inform them that you "regret that you are unable to hire them at this time," however that you would like to be able to call them in the future when another PCA is needed.

27. Training and Ongoing Management

It is essential that everyone who uses PCA help, and who is capable of managing, be able to train those assistants and manage them on a day-to-day, ongoing basis.

This essential need applies equally to those who directly employ PCAs and to those who use agency-employed help. In addition, PCAs with extensive previous training and work experience need your training as well as those with no previous experience.

> Just as a building contractor requires blueprints before ordering lumber, you should organize your needs for assistance & skills before trying to train & manage PCAs

Regardless of who employs a PCA or the PCA's degree of work experience, each and every PCA who assists you will turn to you on the first day of work and ask for the following key information which is available nowhere else:

"Please tell me what specific needs you have for help, as well as how and on what schedule you would like that help provided."

From that point onward, you need training and management skills. There are 4 primary factors to training and managing PCAs:

1) Identify, adopt, and use the qualities and strategies of a good manager

2) Become organized with a list of your needs for assistance, a schedule for those needs, and a list of preferred, safe methods for assisting those needs

3) Provide each PCA with clear initial training instructions, and

4) Provide each PCA with good ongoing management

Training and Ongoing Management

1) Identify, adopt, and use the qualities and strategies of a good manager. Becoming a good trainer and manager is perhaps 75% preparation before the first PCA begins to assist you. Sections I and II of this book address this very important preparation.

Key topics which you might wish to review from these beginning chapters include:

- Observing the human rights which both you and the PCA have
- Understanding the importance, or freedoms, of directly managing the PCAs who assist you
- Determining your appropriate management role by identifying which of the 3 management situations applies to you
- Understanding and respecting why PCAs often quit their jobs and why they are commonly fired, so that you can avoid these management problems
- Knowing how to appropriately use PCA help in various settings
- Knowing about the different types of PCA help which are available, and your role in using each type
- Identifying, adopting, and using the qualities and strategies of a good manager
- Choosing an assertive communication style and avoiding styles which are either weakly passive or abusively aggressive
- Knowing which expectations to have of each PCA, and which expectations they can have of you as their manager, and
- Determining how to provide a pleasant, work-efficient environment with adequate supplies

2) Become organized. It is equally ridiculous for you to attempt to interview and train PCAs before organizing the PCA duties, as it is for a building contractor to order truckloads of lumber and concrete before drawing up a future building's blueprints.

To help you become organized about your needs for assistance and how that assistance should be provided, we suggest that you review sections III and IV of this book.

Topics include:

■ How to avoid abusing PCAs with inappropriate requests for help
■ Making a master list and schedule of your needs for assistance
■ Dividing numerous needs with more than one PCA
■ Identifying various methods for paying PCAs
■ Deciding on a salary rate, and
■ Knowing your tax obligations as an employer

3) Providing clear initial training instructions. There is a number of factors which make teaching easier for you and learning easier for the new PCA:

(a) Be yourself and be pleasant. Don't think of yourself all of a sudden as a supervisor, boss, or employer who must command respect. Instead, consider the new PCA as a friendly individual who is probably quite nervous about the first few times of helping you. Think of her as a teammate.

(b) Speak clearly and not too fast. The objective in teaching is to have someone learn something by the teacher transferring knowledge to the student. That transfer cannot take place if the teacher mumbles, doesn't explain things well, or tries to teach material so fast and in such a rush that the student falls behind in understanding, memorizing, and learning the material.

(c) Give clear, step-by-step instructions. Before you begin teaching, be sure your routine follows an order which is both logical and efficient for your PCA to follow. Logical means that each step of your routine logically leads to the next. Efficient means that the steps of the routine don't waste time or energy of the PCA. In short, you have designed the routine to get all of your needs met while making the routine as easy as possible for the PCA.

(d) Be patient, tolerant, and understanding of mistakes. When anyone is learning something, and even afterward, they can be expected to make mistakes. You should tolerate honestly-made mistakes, however you should assertively state your concern over mistakes which result from a lack of caring about the job.

During this time, the orientation role of the new PCA is comprised of a two-step process. First, they need sufficient time to learn from your training which duties are required and the methods and schedule by which those duties should be performed. Second, they need enough time to develop the habits of performing these duties in an efficient and high quality manner.

Your orientation role during this period is to train the PCA in a manner which will make learning easy and to patiently tolerate the expected mistakes which are certain to occur.

When your new or current PCA makes a mistake, don't be surprised and therefore don't act surprised or become mad. Assure them that making a reasonable number of mistakes is OK and then suggest (if necessary) how the problem can be avoided in the future.

(e) Invite and encourage questions at all times. An essential part of learning is for a student to be able to ask questions about what is not understood. When someone feels free to interrupt your instruction and ask questions, they learn faster -- and that's the objective of teaching. Remember also that there is no such thing as a stupid question, as long as it is a sincere question. A PCA should not be made to feel stupid or foolish for asking a question.

> Make the new PCA comfortable -- be patient of mistakes, show appreciation for duties which are performed well, & stop your instruction as soon as it is no longer needed

(f) Be consistent each time you perform your routine in the order of steps and the way each is performed. No one in a history class could remember how the events of world history occurred if the teacher kept switching around the order of the events and dates. Your own routine will be impossible to learn unless you follow the same order of steps each day.

(g) Do not allow a PCA to perform a duty in the wrong way. A PCA quickly gets into the habit of performing steps of your routine in a certain way. Be sure that they are performing items the correct way from the beginning. It might take no more energy to do something correctly than to do it incorrectly, however it takes much more energy to break a bad habit and re-learn the correct method for performing a task. Do yourself and the PCA a favor -- insist that they "do it right the first time."

(h) Be clear in establishing time schedules. Be clear in telling the PCA about essential times to begin and end your routines. This does not mean dictating the start and stop time for each 3-minute step of your routine. It does mean that you are clear about when you want your PCA to arrive each day and by what time you need certain duties performed so that you, in turn, can meet your daily schedule of appointments, meetings, and activities.

(i) Explain why you prefer a certain order for the steps in your routine, certain methods for each task, and the time schedule for your routine. A PCA will be more interested in respecting your preferences if they understand the reasons why they are important to you and the negative consequences of not respecting the preferences. The negative consequences should not be expressed in terms of "do this task this way or you will be fired," but instead in terms of negative effects on your safety, daily schedule, or increased difficulty for the PCA. Many employees classically grumble about the fact that "they don't understand why they are asked to do things in a certain way." Help the PCA realize why your preferences are important and they will try harder to satisfy those preferences.

(j) Show appreciation for duties which the PCA has learned and is performing well. One of the steps in earning your PCA's respect is to first show them respect and appreciation. In return, they will want to please you by performing your routine in a satisfactory manner. Showing someone appreciation for doing a good job can be much more powerful than even salary in keeping an employee happy. Some volunteers are faithful and loyal to their duties for years, not because of salary but because of appreciation which they receive. Give your PCAs both a salary and appreciation.

(k) While a clear explanation is a good teaching tool, an explanation and a demonstration are even better. The best textbooks and instruction manuals are loaded with diagrams and pictures; a good classroom instructor uses visual aids and handouts. People learn faster when they both hear instruction and see it demonstrated. A picture is truly worth a thousand words, especially if someone is trying to memorize and learn a routine. The quickest way for a new PCA to learn your routine is to hear you narrate the "what and whys" while watching your current PCA perform your routine with you.

The actual teaching of a new PCA will probably take place in one of 2 ways:

a) You verbally direct a new PCA, with no one else present, through the step-by-step procedures of your routine. She must visualize and then perform each duty from your verbal descriptions, at first like a mechanical robot until she begins to memorize the steps and their logical order. Gradually, she performs more and more steps from her memory without verbal prompts or the need for supervision from you. Your instruction should stop as soon as it is no longer needed.

or

b) During the first time that the new PCA sees your routine, ask the newly hired PCA to watch your current PCA perform the routine. While your current PCA performs your routine with you, you should narrate what the PCA is doing and why it is necessary to do it this way. While your current PCA performs your routine and you narrate the whats and whys, have the recruit occasionally participate. This partial participation will make the session more interesting for the new PCA (and she will pay more attention to learning the routine) and it will make the new PCA feel easier next time about performing duties with you on her own.

For the second time, have the new PCA perform practically all of the duties on her own. Narrate what must be done only when the new PCA appears to be "stuck" for remembering the next detail. The more she can do from memory without prompts, the faster she will memorize your routine. You might decide to perform this second session alone with the new PCA, or you might decide to ask your current PCA to standby in the background in case you request an additional demonstration of a certain detail. Unless you are unable to readily communicate and consequently train, you should be sure that you -- and not your current PCA -- is providing the overall instruction; this factor is important for establishing your authority with the new PCA.

In either of these 2 situations, the new PCA will be understandably nervous, so be comforting, patient, and tolerant of mistakes. Be appropriately enthusiastic and quick to give sincere compliments and appreciation when duties are performed correctly.

4) Provide good on-going management once the new PCA has learned the routine. To this point, our first 3 steps have been to identify and use qualities of a good manager, to become organized regarding our needs for PCA assistance, and to provide clear training instructions which are delivered in a favorable manner.

This 4th step involves ongoing management of 4 basic parts.

a) Routinely show appreciation for correctly performed job duties and desirable personal habits. Appreciation serves two purposes: first, to speed the learning process and reinforce high quality work, by praising the PCA when they perform duties correctly, and second, to keep the PCA happy with the job in the long run, by creating a job environment which the PCA likes. More details are contained in the chapter of this book entitled "Methods for Paying PCAs -- Strategies for Expressing Appreciation."

b) Routinely correct poor job performance and personal habits quickly. Don't let poor performance and habits become firmly established. Speak with the PCA about problems in a clear, direct assertive manner. For details

Training and Ongoing Management 311

about assertive communication skills, see the chapter "Passive, Aggressive, and Assertive."

c) Provide a minimum amount of supervision and reminders of task details. No employee likes unnecessarily tight and constant supervision while they are adequately performing duties which have been learned. A very desirable PCA is one who remembers the details of each task and completes them without being reminded. You can encourage this to happen first by supervising and reminding only when necessary, and second by expressing appreciation when the PCA remembers details on their own.

For special, non-routine tasks, clearly explain what you want done, how you want it done, and (if necessary) by when it should be done...and then leave the PCA alone to do the work (if the type of task does not personally involve you). As you leave the area, invite the PCA to call you if any questions or problems develop, or at the time that they finish the task. In the meantime, if you suspect that problems are occurring, peek into the PCA's work area as subtly as possible, as if you are "just stopping by" and not intending to provide "heavy supervision." This softer, non-threatening approach can be reinforced with a short, friendly phrase such as "I just wanted to know if everything is OK."

d) Recognize an employee who states or shows that she no longer wants the job, and part ways with her in a manner which is appropriate to the situation.

It was once said that trying to keep a dying romance alive is like trying to re-heat and eat cold mashed potatoes...no matter how much you try, the results won't be what you had hoped for. The same holds true for trying to keep alive a failing PCA relationship. There are several strategies which you can employ to prevent some upcoming failures from occurring, but once an employer-employee relationship is truly failing, the process is usually irreversable.

If a PCA wants "out," then don't try to barricade the exit door to prevent them from resigning. At other times, you will owe it to your sanity and quality of care to fire a PCA.

Details about attempting to prevent failures as well as actually parting ways are discussed in the chapter "Parting Ways with a PCA."

Of course there is much more to the comprehensive skills of training and management than the comparatively brief outline presented here. However, when the information of this topic is combined with the earlier topics of this book, you will have a quite solid foundation for the purposes of training and managing the PCAs who assist you.

28. Predicting, Recognizing, & Resolving PCA Problems

This chapter looks at ways to remedy both the small, occasional performance problems as well as the larger, chronic problems which can affect the entire relationship between an employer and a PCA employee. The objective is to remedy problems early and keep good PCAs satisfied with their work.

Correcting Simple Performance Problems

Let's begin by looking at the concern which a high quality manager shows each day for keeping employees happy and positively reinforcing, or complimenting, them on their satisfactory work.

In a previous chapter, we examined the importance of paying employees with two types of salaries. In addition to the monetary salary of a weekly paycheck, every worker looks forward to and requires routine doses of genuine appreciation. We won't repeat the reasons why appreciation is so important, or the various ways to express it to a worker, however we will confirm here that routinely shown appreciation is probably the single, most important strategy for keeping a PCA happy with her job.

In addition to keeping workers happy during the "good times" when their work is favorable, regular appreciation also builds a good foundation for any "rocky times" which are certain to occur when their work becomes unsatisfactory and requires correction.

> Showing a PCA appreciation during "good times" will make the PCA more willing to correct bad habits during "bad times"

If an employer or manager rarely speaks to a worker unless something is wrong, then the worker quickly builds a solid association between the approach or conversation from a manager and an upcoming reprimand -- the manager quickly acquires the image which the school principal had during our school days. When Mrs. Unger directed a student "to report to the principal's office," there was little question that the visit would not be pleasant. Why? Because the only association most students traditionally had with the school principal was for corrective discipline...a student was never "sent to see Mr. B." so that he could tell the student how pleased he was with the student's work! Consequently, few of us ever listened openly to the school principal, had much desire to be around him, took his advice very sincerely, or had much desire to be his friend (beyond pleasing him on the surface in order to stay out of trouble).

A PCA manager can choose between assuming a negative "school principal" image or a positive "understanding, caring supervisor" image.

When appreciation is routinely expressed to PCAs, their attitude toward liking their job is significantly increased during good times. In addition, a steady track record of appreciation makes the inevitable rocky times, when an employee's poor performance must be corrected, easier for both parties to accept:

■ First, the PCA likes the employer and the job, and therefore is interested in quickly correcting unsatisfactory performance in order to return to the "good times."

■ Second, the PCA who has been shown appreciation doesn't "shut down" and become instantly defensive when a manager approaches or seems about to bring up some serious discussion. Consequently, this PCA carefully listens and better accepts whatever the manager discusses -- including criticism of performance.

■ Third, when the PCA does receive clear, direct, assertively stated performance problems, he realizes that if his performance is corrected the routine appreciation will begin again and the desired "good times" will resume.

When a PCA's work is satisfactory in an overall sense, but she is not performing a duty in the manner which you prefer or has become sloppy in developing bad habits, the following procedural tips toward quickly correcting bad performance should help:

Predicting, Recognizing, & Resolving PCA Problems   315

1) In advance of these "rocky times," routinely show genuine and appropriate appreciation for those duties which the PCA performs correctly. Further tips on showing appreciation are provided in the chapter, "Paying PCAs: Appreciation & Salary."

2) When performance needs correction, first recognize that "correction" is your true objective, and not discipline, punishment, "showing who's boss," wielding power, or getting-even. Correction should result in changing the way a duty is performed to the correct way, and then resuming appreciation.

> You should spot early warnings of a PCA's job dissatisfaction & correct problems promptly; the PCA often will not complain about problems until it is too late

3) When performance needs correction, be prompt in stating the problem as well as give clear instructions regarding the desired remedy. If a performance problem is allowed to continue for a considerable time, the performance becomes a well established habit which becomes increasingly difficult to correct.

4) State the problem and the desired method in a clear, direct, assertive manner which avoids punishing, abusive aggression as well as weak, poorly stated passiveness. More detail is provided in the chapter, "Passive, Aggressive, Assertive: Which Style is Best for Stating Needs?".

5) As soon as the problem is corrected, and proper performance begins, reinforce the correct behavior with appreciation.

6) If the PCA reacts to your assertive approach in a negative manner or refuses to correct a simple performance problem, then start to examine the following symptoms of healthy and unhealthy job relationships. The problem may be bigger than you at first believed.

Signs of a Healthy Job Relationship

It is easy to spot a worker who is happy with her job. The PCA shows healthy signs of not having significant problems with work, the employer, or personal problems. She seems to like the work, enjoy working for you, and has no personal problems which negatively affect work. She shows this healthy relationship with work in the following ways:

a) By arriving at, or a few minutes in advance of, the scheduled arrival time,

b) By arriving with a reasonably pleasant attitude and being friendly and often smiling at you,

c) By showing interest in you, your activities, and health, and showing this by both initiating and participating in friendly discussions with you,

d) By showing interest in performing quality work for you, a desire to please you by doing a good job, by asking for your preferences on ways that you like to have duties performed, and reacting favorably when you show appreciation for her performance of quality work,

e) By being reasonably neat and clean in appearance,

f) By working steadily and seeing duties through to completion,

g) By remembering most details of the duties as well as your preferences in the ways the details are performed,

h) By speaking clearly and making good eye contact with you while performing many duties,

i) By being willing to work until, and occasionally a bit beyond, the scheduled departure time,

j) By often asking, when leaving, whether there is anything else which she can do for you and by showing some degree of enthusiasm for seeing you next time,

k) By faithfully calling you in as much advance as possible when she finds that she will be late in arriving, or will be unable to arrive at all, and

l) By never arriving under the influence of alcohol or drugs

Symptoms of an Unhealthy Job Relationship

It is often more difficult to spot a worker who is unhappy with her job than one who is happy, because the unhappy worker is often very passive about expressing dissatisfaction. The PCA shows negative symptoms of having a problem, and the problem can be related to not liking the job or the employer, or to a personal problem which is not at all related to the job but does affect job performance. She shows this unhealthy outlook in the following ways:

a) By often arriving late, calling in sick, or just not showing up for scheduled work and seeming not to care about any negative consequences of her habits,

b) By frequently arriving with an unpleasant or negative attitude which can range from being unfriendly to arrogant or abusive toward you,

> Some problems can be resolved, and some cannot; when problems cannot be resolved, prepare early for the PCA's probable departure

c) By having little if any interest in you as an individual, and seldom initiating and often refusing to participate in friendly discussion,

d) By having very little interest or pride in performing high quality work for you, caring little whether you are pleased with the quality of work or whether your preferences are being met, and seeming to lose much of the humanistic respect for working with a human individual who has feelings and needs,

e) By often arriving with a sloppy appearance in clothing and an unkept, dirty, greasy, and possibly smelly lack of personal grooming,

f) By working slowly or sporadically with many rest periods and being easily distracted from work by your TV, magazines, or making phone calls,

g) By often rushing to accomplish job duties as quickly as possible with details left unfinished,

h) By mumbling partial communications with you while avoiding eye contact and seemingly not wanting to be near you,

i) By often cutting duties short and attempting to finish and leave before the scheduled departure time,

j) When leaving, by seldom trying to say much beyond a mumbled "See ya...," and seeming to be bothered by the painful thought of the next scheduled arrival for work,

k) By seeming to care very little whether she arrives on time, and giving you little if any advance notice of expected lateness or inability at all to arrive, or

l) By arriving under the influence of drugs or alcohol.

Possible Reasons Behind Negative Symptoms

These unhealthy job symptoms are merely outward signs of an inner problem. The problem may or may not be work related, and may or may not be resolvable. Some common reasons for outward symptoms of an unhealthy relationship with the PCA job can include:

a) The PCA does not like the working conditions or working for you because --

■ You failed to provide a complete list of all of the expected duties at the time the PCA was hired, and you often add new, unexpected duties,

■ You frequently change the listing of the duties or the order in which they are performed,

■ You often change the expected arrival or departure times, and the duties frequently last beyond the scheduled departure time,

■ You have poorly organized the work area and the duties often waste the PCA's time and energy,

■ You are overly critical of the PCA's work and fail to routinely pay the essential dual salary of appreciation and money,

■ You have habits of relating with a negative, aggressive attitude or other poor employer practices which have been detailed earlier in this book

b) The PCA is tired or dissatisfied with the job because

■ He has worked for you for a short period of time, but discovered that he simply doesn't like one or more of the following factors although all of the facts were clearly stated before he took the job

- the personal nature of the work
- the continuous responsibility of the job
- the hours or days of the job
- the salary of the job
- the commuting distance to the job
- the strength or stamina required for the job
- the interference which the job presents to his other desires or responsibilities (personal, family problems, academic studies, career responsibilities, etc.)

■ He has developed health or stamina problems

■ He has found another job which is more desirable (preferred days or hours, closer to home, higher salary, preferred type of work)

■ He has performed the job for a long period of time and has become tired of performing PCA-type work

Steps in Resolving These or Other Problems

There are 2 primary avenues to take when significant problems are causing negative symptoms to appear:

a) To keep the PCA working, if the problem can be corrected, by clearing up the negative symptoms, or

b) To prepare to replace the PCA (by firing him or accepting his resignation), if the problem cannot be corrected and the symptoms are of a type or severity which cannot be tolerated by you.

If the PCA is a good employee and you want to keep him, then watch for the first signs of unhealthy symptoms and take prompt action. The showing of negative symptoms may signal a very brief and insignificant, non-work related problem, and therefore require no action from you other than to be patient and tolerant during the brief period. If, however, the negative symptoms are severe or more than 2 or 3 days in duration, you might be wise to start some subtle inquiry. If the problem behind the symptoms is work related, then the longer the problem is allowed to persist, the closer the PCA will come to an advance-notice or sudden, unannounced quitting...and it's that sudden quitting which you must try to avoid or for which you must prepare yourself.

The objective is to minimize the chances that a PCA will suddenly blow-up from stored up frustrations and quit, and thus leave you just as suddenly without any assistance. If the PCA has become an undesirable and uncorrectable employee, then your goal may be simply to replace the PCA "ASAP" ("as soon as possible"). If the PCA is a good employee, then your goal should be to attempt to remedy the symptom-causing problem. In either case, as a way of early detection of an upcoming crisis, and as a way of maximizing your control over sudden quittings, you should continuously sniff for signs of smoldering problems around each of the PCAs who work for you

Don't rely on a PCA to take the initiative to bring the problem to your attention and to propose possible remedies. In most cases, you will be able to spot the symptoms of a problem before the PCA even realizes that a problem exists, or before the PCA has the courage to speak with you.

Remember that you are attempting to get rid of the problem which is causing the negative symptom, and not to scold or punish the PCA just for outwardly showing negative symptoms. After all, if a patient has increasingly severe headaches, the appropriate remedy for getting rid of the pain is not usually a prescription for increasing strengths of pain killers, but instead to attempt to identify and correct the actual cause of the pain. In other words, if you merely scold a PCA for negative behavior, he may hide his outward, surface behavior from you, however the source of dissatisfaction will still exist and will eventually need attention.

The step-by-step strategy for identifying and resolving problems, hopefully before they cause your PCA to leave, is to:

1) Identify to yourself which unhealthy, negative symptom the PCA is showing,

2) Ask yourself whether this seems to be a short-term personal problem, which is not related to you or the job, or whether it seems to be job related and is therefore a valid concern to you,

3) If the symptom seems to be related to a problem with you or the job, pick a good time to speak with the PCA (when he is rested and not rushed), identify the symptom which you have recently noticed, and ask in a pleasant, helpful tone whether anything is wrong with which you can help,

4) Listen carefully to the PCA's response to determine what, if anything, you can do to assist in relieving the problem,

5) Be sincere in working to change whatever you reasonably can,

6) Remember that some problems simply do not have solutions, and that you will not be able to save each PCA situation,

7) In any case, when negative symptoms persist, start reviewing your backup list of replacement PCAs in case a sudden replacement is necessary.

When PCA Problems Cannot be Resolved, Prepare to Part Ways

If the problem cannot be corrected, and the negative symptoms shown by the PCA are of a type or severity which cannot be tolerated, then the replacement of the PCA probably cannot be avoided. You should begin to plan the process for replacing her. Steps for a smooth transition between parting ways with a PCA and starting with a new replacement are discussed in the next chapter, "Parting Ways from a PCA."

29. Parting Ways from a PCA

No PCA will work for you forever. Some will work for a limited time, and others will work very successfully for several years. Sooner or later, we all must face the situation of preparing to replace a PCA, and then parting ways with the current PCA...hopefully in that order. This chapter will give you the skills to implement that smooth transition.

Depression About a Departing PCA is Common

A PCA's departure is often an emotional time for you. You have usually become comfortable and trusting of the relationship with the current PCA. Consequently, the employment departure of the PCA often results in the same type of depression, however to less of a severity, than that which occurs with the end of any close relationship or the death of someone close.

There is the feeling of loss of a known and somewhat predictable personality, along with the additional uncertainty about the kind of individual the new PCA will be.

> It is common to feel a sense of loss & depression when a PCA stops working for you

This feeling of anxiety is natural and can be expected to occur, to at least some degree, with each PCA departure. It's a feeling of temporary "emptiness" when a source of reliable and trained help is removed. The feeling can be mild or severe, and equally affects new PCA managers as well as seasoned managers of many years.

If we recognize this feeling as chiefly a loss of a reliable source of help, then we can also recognize that a primary strategy for minimizing the feeling is to have reliable replacement help trained and ready to arrive as the former help departs. The feeling of emptiness is considerably more severe if there is no immediate replacement lined up.

We can minimize the depression of losing a current PCA by planning as early as possible to secure a reliable replacement.

The Simple Facts Behind a PCA Departure

There are several common reasons for parting ways with a PCA, and these are detailed in the chapter, "Reasons PCAs Quit & Are Fired." Regardless of the actual reason, the actual parting has to be initiated by one of the two parties -- either:

a) The PCA decides that he no longer wants to work for you, and he resigns, or

b) You decide that you no longer want the PCA to work for you, and you fire him.

In turn, there are two circumstances for which either of these situations can occur:

1) As an advance-scheduled, well-planned departure, or

2) As an abrupt, sudden crisis departure.

Since your requirement for PCA assistance is usually continuous and does not permit interruption, it is wise, whenever possible, to make each PCA departure an advance-scheduled, well-planned event and to avoid the abrupt quittings and firings.

Steps to Accepting the Resignation from a PCA

In most situations, you will know that a PCA is preparing to resign before she does. To minimize the opportunity for sudden quittings, do your best to maintain an open communication each day with each PCA. Ways of communicating with a PCA include routine "small talk" -- asking about the day-to-day personal events which each PCA feels are important to her as well as periodically asking whether she is having any problems or concerns with work of which you might not be aware.

Parting Ways from a PCA

In addition to the open communication, you should be familiar with the Symptoms of Healthy and Unhealthy Job Relationships which were outlined in the previous chapter. Your monitoring of these symptoms, in addition to "small talk/chit-chat" conversations about problems and everyday life concerns, are good indicators to you whether a PCA might be planning -- consciously or not -- to resign. You will usually be able to spot a PCA's decreasing satisfaction with work before she has done so for herself. Your early readings of these indications are key to avoiding sudden, crisis departures by PCAs.

> You will usually know, long before the PCA does, that she is becoming dissatisfied with her job

You will also find that when you ask an obviously dissatisfied PCA whether there is any problem with her work, that she will often deny the possibility and assure you that everything is fine. At other times, the PCA will agree that a problem exists, but will refuse to talk about it.

At any of these times, keep communication lines open by periodically asking in a supportive, friendly tone about any problems with which you might help or about which you should know. Be prepared -- and don't allow yourself to be surprised -- by a PCA who is showing symptoms of discontent, who denies knowing about any existing problems, and who finally identifies to herself the existence of problems and decides to resign.

When a PCA states her desire to resign, ask first whether the reasons or problems behind the resignation are of the type which can be resolved. Usually they will not be resolvable, because the problem has smoldered for sometime and the PCA is now firm in her decision. If, when you ask for the reason for the resignation, you are given some excuse which doesn't make much logical sense, it is probably futile to attempt to dispute the problem in an effort to save the work relationship...the PCA wants to get out.

In the previous chapter, you saw a list of Symptoms of an Unhealthy Job Relationship, and perhaps you concluded that your current PCA is dissatisfied with her job. You were smart in starting immediately to prepare yourself for a probable, upcoming resignation, and now you are best to accept the actual resignation calmly and with a smile, however difficult that is to do. Do your best not to get outwardly mad and cause the resigning PCA to get mad at you. Remember that a key strategy to avoiding interruptions to your need for continuous PCA assistance is to avoid the abrupt, sudden crisis quittings or firings. Making the PCA mad at you can only serve to increase her desire to leave sooner.

Instead of getting angry, tell the PCA how much you have appreciated her work and how much you regret her resignation (if, indeed, such is the case). Explain that the process of recruiting, interviewing, and hiring a replacement can be a lengthy one. Ask if you may depend upon her assistance for at least 2 (3 or 4?) weeks until you can find that replacement. If you have treated the PCA fairly, and the PCA is not facing a personal crisis which dictates that she leave you immediately, then she will often consent to a reasonable time of continued help to you.

Your responsibility then is to carryout plans which were reviewed in a previous chapter on "Finding PCA Replacements." You need to develop a recruiting strategy, to work steadily on finding the replacement, and to keep the resigning PCA continually updated on your efforts.

Steps to Firing a PCA

A manager will encounter few duties which are as emotionally difficult as firing an employee. The duty is sufficiently difficult that a few managers will even resort to "making life so miserable for an employee that they will quit" as a substitute for firing the employee. This is the cowardly route to take and signifies a poor, weak manager.

Though firing an employee cannot be made easy, the difficulty can be minimized by knowing some basic procedural "dos" and "don'ts."

As mentioned before, there are 2 circumstances within which a PCA can quit or be fired:

1) As an advance-scheduled, well-planned departure, or

2) As an abrupt, sudden crisis departure.

And once more, since your requirement for PCA assistance is usually continuous and does not permit interruption, it is wise to make each PCA parting an advance-scheduled, well-planned event and to avoid the abrupt quittings and firings whenever possible.

There are, however, some situations when a sudden, crisis firing is appropriate. These include any violent or potentially violent situations involving physical abuse, sexual abuse, abuse or carelessness because of heavy use of drugs or alcohol, or any other situations which provide immediate danger to your health, safety, or possessions. It is rare that these will occur between you and a PCA, however know that if any do occur you are justified in a sudden firing.

> Never fire a PCA on impulse while you are mad; the rationale for a valid firing is a clear list of well-established problems which cannot be resolved

It is very rare that you should ever fire a PCA during a time when you are emotionally upset. The firing of a PCA should almost always be carefully planned.

1) When you are tempted to fire a PCA, go off by yourself for a while and do the following:

   a) Ask yourself for a list of reasons for wanting to fire the PCA ("I just hate his guts" is not appropriate; ask yourself for a list of reasons why you feel that way).

   b) Ask yourself whether these reasons or problems can be resolved or whether they therefore truly warrant a firing.

   c) Ask yourself whether the non-resolvable reasons are of a type and severity which you truly cannot tolerate or whether they are just based on a difference in personality styles.

2) After these decisions are made, if circumstances possibly permit, wait at least 24 hours ("sleep on your decision") and review your answers to the questions in step # 1. This helps to cool tendencies toward firings which are unwarranted and based on your emotional impulses. If, however, the problems are of a valid, well-established, long-standing nature, the valid rationale for the upcoming PCA firing will easily endure a 24 hour wait.

3) If your 2 or 3 reviews indicate that a firing is still warranted, it is wise to begin at least mental planning for the replacement PCA before the actual firing. Review the previous chapter on "Finding PCA Replacements" and decide which methods and resources you will use as well as how long the process will take.

4) If possible without your current PCA's knowledge, at least begin the process of recruiting, interviewing, and hiring the replacement PCA before you fire your current PCA.

5) If your decision is firmly and rationally based on valid reasons, then go forcefully ahead with your plans and do not allow yourself to back down:

> a) Perform the firing at the end of the PCA's shift in order to minimize negative situations from the PCA during her assistance to you.
>
> b) Perform the firing without the additional embarrassment to the PCA of having others present, unless you believe that the PCA might be the type to become physically abusive upon hearing the news.
>
> c) Before the PCA arrives on the day of the firing, firmly review the list of reasons which have made the firing absolutely necessary and possibly write out the list if you fear that your mind might go blank during the upcoming confrontation. Many folks actually practice their verbal delivery of the firing several times while alone and facing a mirror.
>
> d) Convince yourself that you will not give the PCA a 2nd chance regardless of excuses, whining, or anger which you may hear. If you have given the matter very careful

thought then you have probably considered and dismissed any reasons why the PCA should not be fired.

e) When addressing the PCA:

- Introduce your need to speak with her and ask her to sit down, "Mary, I would like to speak with you for a minute...please have a seat."

- Position yourself squarely in front of her, face her, make good eye contact with her face and eyes, speak clearly, and use a firm and caring, but not loud or arrogant tone of voice.

Do not begin your delivery with an apology -- you will be doing nothing for which you should be sorry. On the contrary, you will probably be glad and relieved when the task is over...and perhaps the PCA will also feel that way!

> Firing an employee is not easy for anyone; most people practice their phrasing and delivery before meeting with the PCA

- Give straight, honest, and well known reasons as the clear rationale for the firing. Make this presentation clear, brief, and to the point, "Mary, for sometime now you have been coming to work late, either drunk or stoned, and you have almost dropped me twice in performing transfers. The situation is getting steadily worse."

- Before the PCA can reply to these reasons, follow this statement of rationale with a firm, unemotional statement of actual firing. Without this statement, the PCA will think you are just complaining and won't understand that she is being fired. The statement of firing can be stated several different ways, "Mary, based on these reasons -- I believe it's best if we part ways/I have decided to dismiss you/I have decided to replace you/I have decided that I will no longer need your help/I will no longer be asking you to help me/I have decided to let you go/I'm firing you."

- Following this statement of firing, clearly indicate whether the firing is effective immediately ("Mary, please consider this your last day. I will send you your final paycheck tomorrow"), whether you are giving the PCA a period of time to find new employment ("Mary, if you wish I will be glad to keep you for up to two weeks until you find new employment"), or whether you are requesting the PCA to stay a specific amount of time to help while you find and train a replacement ("Mary, I would appreciate your working for 2 more weeks while I find and train a replacement. This will also give you time to find another job.")

- Do not allow yourself to be drawn into an argument or to defensively react to any arrogant or nasty comments from the PCA. Keep a straight, firm, and pleasant face, and if a reply to a nasty response is required many managers simply state (and perhaps have to repeat) "Mary, I'm sorry (or regret) that you feel that way."

- Be sure to collect any house keys or borrowed items at an appropriate time. If the PCA refuses to return keys and you feel that your safety or possessions are threatened, promptly call a locksmith and have your key cores changed.

While it is not uncommon for a fired PCA to become defensive or angry on hearing the news, some other PCAs will actually be relieved and pleased. If a work relationship has become steadily worse, then the work has become a strongly negative situation for both of you. It is surprisingly common for a PCA to thank you for firing him. He might even state that he is relieved because you had the courage to fire him, since he lacked the courage to simply quit. Both of you realize relief after you have finally ended the unpleasant situation.

30. 10 Top Guidelines for Maximum Independent Living

For those of you who have physical limitations and must therefore manage physical assistance from others, this handbook has provided information for living more independently. Even though you might require physical assistance from others, you can still live with a high degree of overall independence.

"Independence" is defined, in part, by "being not subject to control from others." The primary objective of this book has been to put you -- the actual recipient of PCA help -- in control of those who help you...and to avoid having your daily schedule, choice of daily activities and lifestyle, health, safety, and personal freedom controlled by PCAs.

Each of us must take responsibility for shaping our own future -- no one else will do it for us.

This reality should be the driving force behind anyone who wants to control his own life, as each of us should be doing. The very positive consequences of your being in control of your own life, and the depressing negative consequences of allowing others to control you, are summed up in this quote:

> I believe that *we are who we choose to be.*
> Nobody is going to come and save you. You've got to save yourself.
> Nobody is going to give you anything. You've got to go out and fight for it.
> Nobody knows what you want except you, and nobody will be as sorry as you if you don't get it.
> So don't give up you dreams. *

I am often asked during individual counseling sessions as well as large-group lectures, "Would you please list and briefly discuss the key factors which you believe contribute to living independently."

----

* Please see acknowledgement page for source of quote

Usually, before I present my own list, I reverse the question and ask for the opinion of the audience. This both prompts folks to participate in the topic and results in comments which have contributed considerably to the list which I can then pass onto others.

Here, then, is my current "10 top guidelines to maximum independent living" (in no particular order):

1) Become and remain interested and active in a variety of life activities.

Remember that you will get out of life only as much as you put into it. It has also been said that happiness, for many people, "is having something to love, something to do, and a goal for the future."

Get busy and involved in life...education, career, hobbies, leisure, exercise and recreation, and perhaps some sort of spiritual or religious belief. As the saying goes, it is better to wear out (by being active) than to burn out (by going too fast) or to rust out (by doing nothing).

Don't make the classic mistake of passively giving up on an active life and letting your brain turn to mush. You were born with curiosity, imagination, motivation, the ability to think and problem-solve, and the ability to laugh and be reasonably happy. If you don't use these abilities, you will surely lose them.

> I believe that *we are who we choose to be.* *

Your physical limitations have no relationship to your ability to be active and happy. If you choose a lifetime of decreasing interest and activity in the life going on around you, you will become physically unhealthy and psychologically depressed. Your eventual death will be a lonely one, for few people will find you interesting, and therefore few will routinely want your company.

2) Develop a lifestyle habit of "preventative preparation and maintenance" toward health and essential supplies.

You are probably quite dependent upon certain medications, medical supplies, and devices and equipment which accommodate your physical limitations. Supplies will run out as you consume them, devices and equipment will break down and wear out as you use them, and your personal health will be minimized by sickness from time to time.

One of the keys to independent living is to minimze your inactive "down time" that is due to sickness or the lack of supplies or equipment upon which you are dependent. Therefore one of your lifetime goals is to prevent any foreseeable, predictable down time from occurring, even though a much smaller amount of inactivity will still occur from problems which are completely unpredictable.

Make a habit of periodically checking your level of supplies and re-ordering in advance of running out of any item. Make a habit of inspecting and listening to mechanical equipment for tell-tale, early signs of wear, and repair or replace parts or entire items before inconvenient wear-outs and breakdowns happen.

For more details on this topic, see the chapter "The Favorable Physical Work Environment."

3) Become the best one-source reference on your own medical history.

Car buffs, who love their cars and want to keep them in tip-top shape, are quick to learn at least the basics about how their car functions, what parts typically breakdown, how to perform maintenance to prevent most breakdowns, and what to do when breakdowns do happen. These folks also keep records about what breakdowns have occurred and what repairs were performed to remedy the problems. After all, when problems happen in the future and the car owner consults a mechanic for repairs, the mechanic will usually ask the owner whether this problem has happened before and what repairs were made.

If a car buff takes these steps to keep his car in good running order, shouldn't you do at least as much to keep your own body in good running order?

> Nobody is going to come and save you. You've got to save yourself. *

To maximize your own good health, and minimize the times of poor health, you should take responsibility for coordinating your own health care. You cannot expect anyone else to care as much about your body as you should...and you cannot expect anyone else to do this for you.

If you know enough about your body's medical history and how to care for it, you will know which self-care steps to take when some illnesses and emergencies occur. When more complex problems happen, your ability to provide information about your medical background will be very helpful to medical authorities whom you consult.

Learn everything which you reasonably can about --

- how your body functions
- how your disability affects those functions
- which body functions are most prone to malfunction or sickness
- what to do when common sicknesses occur

In addition, keep mental or written records of dates and details about --

- which major illnesses you have had
- the treatment and medications used to combat each illness

More details about this topic are found in the chapters "Settings in Which You Use Help" and "Types of Help & the Services Each Performs."

4) Remember that medical authorities are your employees, and they should be consulted by you whenever you have questions about your responsibility to coordinate your own health care.

The days are over for fearing the authority of medical professionals and following their orders without asking questions. Most of today's professionals welcome a patient who asks sincere questions and participates in decisions about diagnoses, treatments, medications, and self-care.

Do not fear the possible anger of health professionals in response to questions which you have about how your body works, what has gone wrong with it in the past and what might go wrong in the future, and what you should do to maximize your good health. You are directly or indirectly paying these people for their services, and that makes them your employees!

> Nobody is going to give you anything. You've got to go out and fight for it. *

If you have sincere questions, you have the ethical and legal rights to ask them and get answers which you understand. If your medical professional doesn't respect those rights, then you should change professionals (you have the right to do that also).

More details about this topic are found in the chapters "Settings in Which You Use Help" and "Types of Help & the Services Each Performs."

5) Use a clear, direct, assertive style of communication with others, and avoid communication which is either weakly passive or abusively aggressive.

Remember that others cannot possibly be responsible for accommodating your needs which they do not know about. It is your responsibility to make your needs known in a way which is clear and direct. You should avoid communication which is weakly passive and communicates only partial messages, or abusively aggressive and assaults and offends people. These people can include parents, relatives, a spouse, friends, co-workers, and medical professionals.

For more detail on this topic, see the chapter "Assertive, Passive, and Aggressive...Which Style is Best for Stating my Needs?"

6) Be persistent in resolving problems and achieving goals.

> Nobody knows what you want except you, and nobody will be as sorry as you if you don't get it. *

Those who enjoy living independently are not always very intelligent...there are many independent and successful folks who make lots of mistakes and have little formal education. They are not always wealthy...most who live independently work very hard for a living. They are not always those with a large family or a ready staff of "helpers" nearby to provide assistance...many achievers simply know how to find and tap the resources existing around them.

However, those who live independently do have at least one common trait...they are all persistent in achieving what they need or want.

Perhaps your current goals include getting a college education, landing a job, living in your own apartment or house, getting a wheelchair repaired, or suddenly finding a new PCA. Seldom is the path which leads to a goal as simple and problem-free as it at first seemed. Additional problems appear, finances run short, or perhaps personal sickness erupts.

The key to achieving your goals is persistence...not giving up.

Being persistent begins with being sufficiently flexible in life to enable "riding out," or coping with unexpected obstacles which appear between you and a goal. "Moguls" ("moe-gulls") are the sudden bumps that a skier encounters as he skis down a snowy mountainside. If he keeps his knees stiff and not flexible, he will tumble and fall at the first mogul he meets. If, on the other hand, he keeps his knees bent and flexible, he can better cope with sudden obstacles in his path.

As you go through life and pursue various goals, keep your knees bent and be flexible to obstacles and the need to compromise or change personal plans. When unexpected barriers do appear -- or you tumble and fall -- be persistent, get back up, and find a new path to your goal.

7) Take responsibility for your own on-going health, and realize that you, alone, are responsible for your total well-being.

In a hospital or rehabilitation center, it becomes easy to assume that physicians, therapists, and nurses are legally responsible for your care and well-being. Upon discharge, it is equally easy to assume that your parents, relatives, spouse, or home health aide are now responsible for maintaining your health and providing physical assistance for your needs.

No matter how much a loved one "loves and cares for you," it is seldom appropriate for you to transfer to them the on-going responsibility for your own well-being.

If you are psychologically capable of coordinating your own care and needs, then you are ethically responsible for doing so. And if you are capable of coordinating your own care, you are very fortunate because, as a well-known song-writer once said, "No one will ever care for you as much as you can...or should."

For more details on this topic, see the chapters "Why Should You Learn to Manage the Help You Use?" and "The 3 Management Situations: Which Applies to You?"

8) Take responsibility for your own on-going rehabilitation, and realize that rehabilitation is a life-long process.

If we define rehabilitation simply as "accommodating limitations to enable leading as full a life as you wish," then it is obvious that the rehabilitative process does not end -- but just begins -- with discharge from a medical facility.

Your health and physical abilities and disabilities will be constantly changing throughout your lifetime. Consequently, it will be up to you to devise new ways to accommodate new limitations, or to become progressively inactive as each new limitation occurs.

While you are an in-patient at a medical facility, tap the expertise of the professionals around you for ideas on accommodating your limitations. During your lifetime after discharge, combine consultations with those pros with your own creativity in order to design new accommodations as necessary.

More details about this topic are found in the chapters "Settings in Which You Use Help" and "Types of Help & the Services Each Performs."

9) Develop a list of local and national resources and use them to quickly obtain goods and services as needed.

An important initial step in resolving many types of problems is knowing where to find help.

That help might come in the form of services or tangible goods. Services can include advice, counseling, medical treatment, home health aide assistance, and repairs to various devices and equipment. Tangible goods can include any physical item which is loaned, rented, or purchased from a store or similar facility. These goods could be library books, medications, medical equipment and repair parts, household supplies, food, or clothing.

There are almost as many ways to find resources as there are resources, themselves. The 3 most common paths are asking friends or authorities for referrals, consulting a telephone yellow pages, and looking through specialized directories which list contact details.

When you encounter the need for a specific service or tangible good, be assured that there is usually a resource which will supply it to you. Get cracking, find a supplier, and resolve your problem.

10) If you are dependent on physical assistance for certain personal needs, learn how to manage and be in control of those who assist you.

As outlined in the beginning of this chapter, living independently is living free from the control of others. You must be free to choose your own daily schedule and activities, and to coordinate any necessary physical assistance to realize that lifestyle.

This book is by far the single, most comprehensive reference which teaches you how to be in control of that help that you use or employ.

So don't give up your dreams! *

Your Personal Management Notes: What Has Worked for You and What Has Not

Your Personal Management Notes

How to Order Copies of this Book

Single and multiple-copy orders are welcome by mail (no phone orders or inquiries, please) at the address below. This text is well structured for classroom and group instruction, and the discounts available for multi-copy orders are listed below.
Payment:
■ All orders must be accompanied by prepayment in U.S. funds. We regret that we cannot accept cash, credit card, or COD orders.
■ All personal, non-agency orders must be prepaid by personal check, bank check, or money order. Orders with bank checks or MOs are usually shipped within 5 working days of our receipt; orders with personal checks are shipped as soon as the check clears, usually within 3 weeks.
■ Agency and institutional orders may also be prepaid by check. POs are accepted for <u>multiple-copy</u> orders when fully detailed and signed. PO payment terms are 30 days net.
Costs:
■ Single copy	$18.95 (+$2 Postage & Handling)
■ Multiple copies	
2-5 copies	18.75 (+$1.85 each)
6-9 copies	18.50 (+$1.60 each)
10-30 copies	17.95 (+$1.50 each)
30+ copies	Please write for special-discount quotation

■ New York State addresses must add their county's sales tax to the purchase price before adding the postal charge. If tax exempt, please include a N.Y.S. certificate with your order.
■ Orders shipped outside of the U.S. should add $3.00 postage per copy to above costs.
■ Send order and prepayment to Saratoga Access Publications, P.O. Box 2346, Clifton Park, NY 12065.
Your order should contain the following details :
■ The "ship to" name, street address, city-state-zip
■ Your phone number, in case we have questions
■ The number of copies you wish
    x   The appropriate per-copy price (see chart above)
    +   N.Y.S. sales tax (if applicable)
    +   Postage & handling (see chart above)
    =   The total of the enclosed prepayment
We would appreciate your comments about this book:
■ Is it helpful to you? How could its next edition be improved? **Thank you!** -- Al De Graff, Author

How to Order Copies of this Book

Single and multiple-copy orders are welcome by mail (no phone orders or inquiries, please) at the address below. This text is well structured for classroom and group instruction, and the discounts available for multi-copy orders are listed below.
Payment:
▪ All orders must be accompanied by prepayment in U.S. funds. We regret that we cannot accept cash, credit card, or COD orders.
▪ All personal, non-agency orders must be prepaid by personal check, bank check, or money order. Orders with bank checks or MOs are usually shipped within 5 working days of our receipt; orders with personal checks are shipped as soon as the check clears, usually within 3 weeks.
▪ Agency and institutional orders may also be prepaid by check. POs are accepted for <u>multiple-copy</u> orders when fully detailed and signed. PO payment terms are 30 days net.
Costs:

▪ Single copy	$18.95 (+$2 Postage & Handling)
▪ Multiple copies	
2-5 copies	18.75 (+$1.85 each)
6-9 copies	18.50 (+$1.60 each)
10-30 copies	17.95 (+$1.50 each)
30+ copies	Please write for special-discount quotation

▪ New York State addresses must add their county's sales tax to the purchase price before adding the postal charge. If tax exempt, please include a N.Y.S. certificate with your order.
▪ Orders shipped outside of the U.S. should add $3.00 postage per copy to above costs.
▪ Send order and prepayment to Saratoga Access Publications, P.O. Box 2346, Clifton Park, NY 12065.
Your order should contain the following details :
▪ The "ship to" name, street address, city-state-zip
▪ Your phone number, in case we have questions
▪ The number of copies you wish
    x   The appropriate per-copy price (see chart above)
    +   N.Y.S. sales tax (if applicable)
    +   Postage & handling (see chart above)
    =   The total of the enclosed prepayment
We would appreciate your comments about this book:
▪ Is it helpful to you? How could its next edition be improved? **Thank you!** -- Al De Graff, Author